Praise for Bill Hayes and Sleep Demons

"What if the hum [of sleep] never comes? That's what writer and photographer Bill Hayes explores in his magnificent book *Sleep Demons*, part reflection on his own lifelong turmoil in the nocturne, part sweeping inquiry into the sometimes converging, sometimes colliding worlds of sleep research, psychology, medicine, mythology, aging, and mental health."
—Maria Popova, *Brain Pickings*

"A skilled and graceful debut that variously reads like a journey of scientific discovery, a personal memoir, and a literary episode of *Ripley's Believe It or Not*. . . . An intelligent, beautifully written book, Hayes's curious hybrid will delight readers who snore past dawn as well as those who pace away while the midnight oil burns."
—*Publishers Weekly* (starred review)

"A graceful hybrid of a book that's half research treatise and half memoir. . . . Lovely writing that may keep readers up late into the evening."
—*Entertainment Weekly*

"Memoir, history, and science come together and apart again in a book that reads very much like a dream, switching genre and subject with a beautiful logic of its own, illuminated now and then with flashes of gorgeous insight. . . . Read this one, savor it, just don't take it to bed with you."
—*Out* magazine

"Hayes has created something that goes beyond mere memoir; call it obsessional autobiography. . . . Hayes' polished writing and fearless revelations make it work beautifully."
—*San Francisco Chronicle*

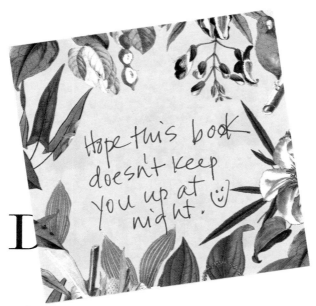

Hope this book
doesn't keep
you up at
night.

L

An Insomniac's Memoir

WITH A NEW PREFACE

Bill Hayes

THE UNIVERSITY OF CHICAGO PRESS

The University of Chicago Press, Chicago 60637
© 2018 by William Hayes
All rights reserved. No part of this book may be used or reproduced in any manner whatsoever without written permission, except in the case of brief quotations in critical articles and reviews. For more information, contact the University of Chicago Press, 1427 E. 60th St., Chicago, IL 60637.
Published 2018
Printed in the United States of America

27 26 25 24 23 22 21 20 19 18   1 2 3 4 5

ISBN-13: 978-0-226-56083-0 (paper)
ISBN-13: 978-0-226-56097-7 (e-book)
DOI: https://doi.org/10.7208/chicago/9780226560977.001.0001

AUTHOR'S NOTES

Some names have been changed in the author's memoir.

Although every attempt has been made to ensure the accuracy of information on sleep disorders herein, this book does not constitute medical advice.

PUBLICATION ACKNOWLEDGMENTS

Sleep Demons was first published by Washington Square Press in 2001. Brief portions of this book were originally published in different forms in the following publications: *Details*, *DoubleTake*, *Mother Jones*, *The New York Times Magazine*, Salon.com, *San Francisco Focus*, and *Speak*.

PERMISSIONS ACKNOWLEDGMENTS

Grateful acknowledgment is made to the following for permission to reprint previously published material:

Farrar, Straus and Giroux, LLC, and Faber and Faber Limited: Excerpt from "The Man with Night Sweats" from *Collected Poems* by Thom Gunn. Copyright © 1994 by Thom Gunn. Reprinted by permission of Farrar, Straus and Giroux, LLC, and Faber and Faber Ltd.

Farrar, Straus and Giroux, LLC, and Weidenfeld & Nicolson: Excerpt from *The White Album* by Joan Didion. Copyright © 1979 by Joan Didion. Reprinted by permission of Farrar, Straus and Giroux, LLC, and Weidenfeld & Nicolson.

Indiana University Press: Excerpt from *Lucretius: The Way Things Are*, translated by Rolfe Humphries, pp. 148–49. Copyright © 1968 by Indiana University Press. Reprinted by permission of Indiana University Press.

Penguin Putnam, Inc., and Penguin Books Limited: Excerpt from "Two Forms of Insomnia" from *Selected Poems* by Jorge Luis Borges. Copyright © 1999 by Alan S. Trueblood. Reprinted by permission of Viking Penguin, a division of Penguin Putnam, Inc., and Penguin Books Ltd.

Philosophical Library, New York: Excerpts from *Sleep* by Marie Carmichael Stopes. Copyright © 1956 by the Philosophical Library. Reprinted by permission of The Philosophical Library, New York.

The University of Chicago Press: Excerpts from *Sleep and Wakefulness* by Nathaniel Kleitman. Copyright © 1939 and 1963 by The University of Chicago. Reprinted by permission of The University of Chicago Press.

Library of Congress Cataloging-in-Publication Data

Names: Hayes, Bill, 1961– author.
Title: Sleep demons : an insomniac's memoir : with a new preface / Bill Hayes.
Description: Chicago : The University of Chicago Press, 2018. |
Includes bibliographical references and index. | Originally published: New York : Washington Square Press, 2001.
Identifiers: LCCN 2017048416 | ISBN 9780226560830 (pbk. : alk. paper) | ISBN 9780226560977 (e-book)
Subjects: LCSH: Hayes, Bill, 1961– | Sleep disorders—Patients—Biography. | Insomniacs—Biography.
Classification: LCC RC548 .H394 2018 | DDC 616.8/498—dc23
LC record available at https://lccn.loc.gov/2017048416

♾ This paper meets the requirements of ANSI/NISO Z39.48-1992 (Permanence of Paper).

For Steve Byrne

CONTENTS

PART THREE: NIGHT SWEATS

Preface, 2017

SLEEP DEMONS, my first book, had its genesis in a single
line that came into my mind on a sleepless night more than
twenty years ago. I was lying awake next to my partner, Steve,
who was as usual snoozing soundly, when finally I'd just had it.
Utterly exasperated, I thought: *I would steal an hour of his sleep
if I could—I'd slip beneath his eyelids and yank it right out of him.*

The writer in me knew the line was too good to risk forgetting, so I got out of bed and wrote it down on a pad in another
room. Over the next few weeks, I expanded upon it and wrote
a short, lyrical essay on insomnia, a condition I had struggled
with since childhood. I was working full-time for a nonprofit in
San Francisco, and I would write in the early mornings or during
those frequent midnight hours when I couldn't sleep. The per-

sonal essay was a form I had chosen partly out of practicality—the short length, one to two thousand words, suited my limited writing time—but also out of admiration for work by writers such as Joan Didion, Susan Sontag, and Montaigne. In fact, I had in mind as a model Didion's essay "In Bed," a piece she'd written about having migraine headaches, as I worked on my essay "The Insomniac."

I had only a few publishing credits to my name when, to my surprise, the *New York Times Magazine* picked my piece out of a slush pile and ran it in their Lives column in July 1996. It struck a chord with fellow insomniacs and drew interest from other magazine editors and a few literary agents. I began to think about the possibility of writing a book, though about what exactly I wasn't sure.

Meanwhile, I still had chronic insomnia, some nights not sleeping at all. My doctor suggested I go to the Sleep Research Center at Stanford University, a clinic founded and made famous by the innovative and ambitious William C. Dement, MD. My exam with one of the center's staff doctors was helpful but not life changing (he basically diagnosed garden-variety anxiety, which could cause an episode of insomnia, which then could escalate rapidly into anxiety about sleeplessness itself).

Far more significant was my visit that same day to the Stanford University bookstore. As I browsed the medical school's shelves, my eyes fell upon two fat volumes: a recently published textbook on treating sleep disorders coedited by Dr. Dement, and an early twentieth-century book by someone named Nathaniel Kleitman with the appealingly plain title *Sleep and Wakefulness*. I remember thinking it would be a stretch financially to buy both books, especially the textbook, but my gut told me I should. As it turned out, they gave me the keys to figuring out how I could write a book on insomnia.

In Kleitman, I found a brilliant, idiosyncratic scientist who had pioneered studies on sleep in the 1930s and '40s and, along with a younger colleague, Eugene Aserinsky, discovered REM sleep. He also wrote precisely, elegantly, almost poetically, about sleep, his obsession—an obsession I shared.

I learned that Dr. Dement had been a protégé of Kleitman's at the University of Chicago. One day while scanning the table of contents of his medical textbook, I had an epiphany. Here I found chapters on every known sleep disorder: somnambulism (sleepwalking), somniloquy (sleeptalking), sleep apnea, narcolepsy, sleep paralysis, varieties of insomnia, and so on. Here, too, was scientific research on the development of sleep in human beings, beginning in utero. In a flash, I saw that I could go beyond insomnia and investigate other sleep disturbances— that this could be a way to organize chapters. And by telling Kleitman's story as well, I could delve into the history of sleep science through one compelling central figure, a sort of foil for me, while weaving in reminiscences of my life and of the personal demons, such as struggling with my sexuality, that had triggered bouts of insomnia over the years.

I soon learned a lesson that many first-time authors do: no one can teach you how to write a book; you have to figure it out in your own way. To keep track of the three interweaving narratives and the various sleep disorders I was covering, I came up with a system of color-coded index cards pinned to a bulletin board. I delivered the manuscript in late 2000, and the book was published the following year, shortly after my fortieth birthday. For the cover, my friend the late Maurice Sendak created an original drawing based on Henry Fuseli's eighteenth-century painting *The Nightmare*; however, in place of the woman splayed on the bed, he drew me.

The book did well critically, though it was published in only one edition, which went out of print more than a decade ago. But I was fortunate in that *Sleep Demons* led to a contract for two additional books, which I structured in a similar way and wrote in fairly quick succession. The first was a natural history of human blood titled *Five Quarts* (the amount of blood in the body), interwoven with a personal narrative dominated by my ground-zero experience of the AIDS epidemic in San Francisco in the 1980s and '90s. The second, *The Anatomist*, tells the story behind the nineteenth-century classic *Gray's Anatomy* while also chronicling my own education in human anatomy, including dissecting cadavers alongside medical students at UCSF.

I now see these three books as a trilogy. I had not planned it that way at the outset. But all three are as closely connected as ligaments are to bones by my fascination with the human body, with medical history, and, more specifically, with figures who played bit parts in the much larger history of science. Henry Gray in *The Anatomist* and Paul Ehrlich in *Five Quarts* are counterparts to Kleitman and Aserinsky in *Sleep Demons*—questing eccentrics who made an impact in their fields but are otherwise largely unknown. As I wrote each book, I had the feeling I was rescuing these medical men from relative obscurity by telling their stories.

But there's another, more personal reason I see the three books as a trilogy: they are very much products of the period during which I wrote them, 1996–2006, and they trace my life over those years chronologically. As I've noted, *Sleep Demons* originated with a single vivid thought about my peacefully sleeping partner. Ten years later, just two weeks after I'd submitted the first draft of *The Anatomist* to my publisher, my partner Steve, with whom I'd lived for almost seventeen years, died unexpectedly of a heart attack in bed beside me. He was only forty-three. (To the initial draft of *The Anatomist*, I later added an epilogue dealing with Steve's death.) This brought an end not just to my life in San Francisco—I subsequently moved to New York—but also to this body of work. Steve had been a constant source of encouragement and inspiration for my writing. Now I was on my own.

With the move to New York, my insomnia—long such a bane

of my existence—unexpectedly changed too, from a demon to, well, something different; not a joy—that would be pushing it too far—but something I simply accepted as part of my nature. (Losing two great loves—my second partner, Oliver Sacks, died of cancer in 2015—has also put losing a few nights' sleep into perspective.) I still don't sleep well. But in New York, which I came to call Insomniac City (the title of my recent memoir), I felt a sense of kinship with others who were awake—which is to say alive—at night. Indeed, in some ways I now view insomnia as the epitome of aliveness, of *wakefulness*, to use one of Kleitman's favored terms. I probably could not write *Sleep Demons* today, but at the same time I'm grateful I had the opportunity to write the book when I did. Yes, this is an insomniac's memoir, a history of sleep research, and a lone scientist's story all combined. But at its heart, *Sleep Demons* is about gaining insight into the complex, often mysterious relationship between two diametrical states of being—wakefulness and sleep:

As with desire, it resists pursuit. Sleep must come find you. Nevertheless, I look for it.

—Bill Hayes, August 2017

PART ONE

WAKEFULNESS

Without wakefulness,
sleep cannot be said to exist.

—Nathaniel Kleitman
Sleep and Wakefulness, 1939

Chapter 1

☙

In Utero

I GREW UP in a family where the question "How'd you sleep?" was a topic of genuine reflection at the breakfast table. My five sisters and I each rated the last night's particular qualities—when we fell asleep, how often we woke, what we dreamed, *if* we dreamed. My father's response influenced the family's mood for the day: if "lousy," the rest of us felt lousy, too. If there's such a thing as an insomnia gene, Dad passed it on to me, along with his green eyes and Irish melancholy.

I lay awake as a young boy, my mind racing like the spell-check function on a computer, scanning all data, lighting on images, moments, fragments of conversation, impossible to turn off. As a sleeping aid, I would try to recall my entire life—a straight narrative from first to last incident—thereby imposing order on the inventory of desire and memory. My story always started with a plane ride from Minneapolis to Spokane—a trip that actually occurred, the recollection of which, however, may be imaginary. I was no older than three. But there I am regardless, in memory as if in a movie, still gazing out the window of a jet.

If my boyhood story didn't lull me to sleep, I'd sneak into the den, where I could find my mother, watching Johnny Carson and drinking Coca-Cola, simultaneously smoking Pall Malls and folding laundry. For her, I suspect, not sleeping offered time on her own. For me, visiting Mom after midnight was the only time I had her to myself in such a big family. She never shooed me back to bed. I helped her fold socks, she gave me a glass of Coke. Some combination of the two helped me fall asleep.

After she had put me to bed, I would occasionally wander back again, sleepwalking. I remembered nothing of these night visits. I learned of them at the breakfast table, next morning, where they were a source of laughter from my sisters that left me uneasy. Thirty years later, my mother still recalls how oddly I acted: I did not sit down with her, didn't speak or respond to her voice. I appeared to be looking for something. Without waking me, she would gently lead me back to my room. This sleep disorder, a "parasomnia" that rarely appears in adults, lasted about two years.

In some ways, I find sleepwalking more perplexing than sleeplessness—perhaps because it afflicted me while I was so young, then let me go, never to return again. If the insomniac is a shadow of his daylight self, existing nightlong on nothing but the fumes of consciousness, then the somnambulist is like an animal whose back leg drags a steel trap—the mind is fleeing and the body is inextricably attached.

Where did I want to go? Out of that house, I imagine.

Away from the person I saw myself becoming. Toward a dreamed-up boy, with a new story, a different version of myself.

Now, halfway through my life, I still wander at night. I still seek the peerless soporific. Everybody has a cure to recommend, whether it's warm milk, frisky sex, or melatonin. One friend solemnly prescribes whiffing dirty socks before turning out the lights. I find, though, that home remedies are no more effective than aphrodisiacs. Sleeping pills can force the body into unconsciousness, it's true. I've had my jags on Halcion and Xanax, Ambien and Restoril. I've slept many times on those delicious, light-blue pillows. But the body is never really tricked. The difference between drugged and natural sleep eventually reveals itself, like the difference between an affair and true romance. It shows up in your eyes. Sleep acts, in this regard, more like an emotion than a bodily function. As with desire, it resists pursuit. Sleep must come find you.

Nevertheless, I look for it. If not my own, then the sleep of others. You might find me on the subway staring as you come out of a snooze. You'd see no guilt on my face for watching so shamelessly, only fascination. When people doze in public, the human animal comes out. They burrow into their own clothing or nestle into a friend's shoulder. Undefended from their own small indiscretions, they scratch, grunt, fart, drool, grit their teeth. People know this happens and try to hide themselves: they pull down a hat or put on sunglasses; duck under a newspaper or drape an arm over the face. Left exposed, it is as if they're caught naked: a hand instinctively reaches up to shield their eyes, where it often remains until the lids open.

Sleep also has the uncanny ability both to infantilize and to age, which is especially strange to see in the person with whom you are intimate. After a night of insomnia, sometimes I stand at the bedroom door, coffee in hand, watching my partner of ten years, Steve, sleep. One morning, he's curled up in the fetal position, legs tucked up to his chest, arms hugging a pillow. He looks as vulnerable as a baby. With a snort, he rolls onto his back, the planes of his face fall into shadows, and suddenly he's middle-aged. Another morning, Steve sleeps so soundlessly I have to make sure he's still breathing. I tiptoe in and hover over him. I hold my own breath, not making a sound. Yet it is as if his sleeping self recognizes me—it vanishes in a heartbeat. He wakes up, startled, wondering what the hell I'm doing.

Sleep scientists spend their entire waking lives engaged in this kind of surveillance. They may stay up all night just to watch someone awaken. They treat bizarre and dangerous disorders—narcolepsy, obstructive sleep apnea, African sleeping sickness, fatal familial insomnia—as well as the everyday sleep disturbances of people like me. I've looked into their findings, in search of answers that my own body refuses to divulge. I've studied the work of early sleep researchers, along with books on anatomy, mythology, mental disorders, aging. While none of what I've learned has fully unraveled the mystery of sleep, least of all in my own life, I have come to see that sleep itself tells a story.

The ancient Greeks envisioned sleep to be Hypnos, the twin brother of death, Thanatos. A minor god, born of Night, Hypnos lived in a dark, underworld cave on the island of Lemnos. The River of Forgetfulness flowed through the cavern where Hypnos lay on pillows surrounded by his many sons, including Morpheus, the dream-bringer. Unlike his twin, Hypnos was considered a friend of mortals, a healer of body and mind. He took different forms as he wandered the earth—a bird or a child, but most often a benevolent warrior carrying a horn, from which he would drip a sleep elixir. The Greeks apparently took his gifts for granted. There were neither temples devoted to Hypnos nor songs to thank him. No cult arose to worship sleep, which seems particularly odd, if not irreverent, for surely there were ancient insomniacs.

A Greek physician named Alcmaeon, from the sixth century B.C., is credited with the first recorded theory on the cause of sleep. He thought it was due to blood vessels of the brain becoming engorged. Aristotle, two hundred years later, viewed sleep as the opposite of wakefulness, one of the *contraries* that "are seen always to present themselves in the same subject, and to be affections of the same: examples are— health and sickness, beauty and ugliness, strength and weakness, sight and blindness, hearing and deafness." In a sense, Aristotle took the Greek myth and recast it: now, sleep was the evil twin of wakefulness. "Sleep," he noted, "is evidently a privation of waking." Basing his theory on personal observation rather than traditional thought, Aristotle concluded that sleep was the result of vapors generated by the digestion of food, which then rose to the brain. The bigger the meal, the greater the vapors, the sleepier one got.

Aristotle's ideas remained influential for centuries. Experts who followed devoted themselves to hunting down sleep to its anatomical root, if only in hope of extending wakefulness. If not in the stomach, then possibly behind the eyes? The thyroid, at the base of the neck, was thought to be a sleep-inducing gland until doctors recognized that removing it did not cause insomnia. Another example—nonsensical in hindsight—can be found in David Hartley's *Observations on Man: His Frame, His Duty, and His Expectations,* published more than two thousand years after Aristotle, in 1749. Inquiring into "the intimate and precise nature of sleep," Hartley, an English doctor, stated that sleep could be explained by the "Doctrine of Vibrations." As he saw it, the human body was like a sack of Jell-O—a jiggling mass of solids and fluids. It must, on occasion, come to rest. To Hartley and his contemporaries, sleep was considered necessary but intrinsically bad. Oversleeping (or, heaven forbid, enjoying sleep) demonstrated a character flaw; it was a symptom of sloth and low intelligence.

By the early twentieth century, proposed theories weren't any more accurate. According to the French scientist Claparède, sleep resulted from a loss of interest in one's surroundings (*réaction de désintérêt*); likewise, one woke up because one tired of sleeping. This "instinct" was thought to serve an essential defensive function: "We sleep not because we are intoxicated or exhausted," Claparède wrote in 1905, "but in order to prevent our becoming intoxicated or exhausted." It was like saying that we breathe in order not to die of asphyxiation, as later scientists pointed out. His theory was related to a prevailing idea that sleep was caused by mysterious toxins in the blood, the "products of wakefulness." Long popular, this "hypnotoxin theory" held that fatigue was a poisonous substance that built up over the day, finally causing sleep at night, at which time it was eliminated. The more you slept, the more you had been bedeviled by the day's toxins.

The notion that we are poisoned and *possessed* by sleep would've made perfect sense to me as a little boy. That's how my parents and sisters appeared when I looked in on them. Awakened by a stomachache or bad dream, I would sometimes scurry down the chilly hall to Mom and Dad's room, two doors away, right after the kids' bathroom. (In our home, where every room conveyed its rank in the family hierarchy, each with its own set of rules, the title "the master bedroom" was especially apt.) Having pushed open their door, I'd pause in the entryway, just past the master bathroom, and peer around the corner toward where they slept.

They had twin beds, pushed together, united by a teakwood headboard and a single quilt. Watching their lumpish figures, like the dark mounds of snow piled at either side of our driveway, I felt scared for a moment. They were there, but not present: faces buried in pillows; breathing raspily; tongues clacking. I stepped forward. Then it was I who scared them. Mom would wake with a sudden gasp—feet on the floor even before she recognized which child stood before her. She'd whisk me back to my room as Dad's figure half-rose in the background. His sleep, we all understood, was not to be disturbed.

I never crawled into bed with them. None of us kids did. But when I was a bit older, ten or eleven, I had to share a bed with my father on occasional weekend ski trips—promoted in advance as "just for the boys." As Dad merrily explained to my sisters, "No squaws allowed."

I was used to sleeping by myself. I can still recall my dread as we got into bed at the ski lodge. Lying on my back, feeling pinioned between the starched sheets, I could hear a transformation take place after Dad said good-night and turned out the lights. Maybe he took a Valium, as he sometimes did at home. His breathing, at first silent, steadily became pronounced. If I turned to face him, I'd be bathed in it, a warm blast of toothpaste and Johnnie Walker. I rolled in the other direction. The room was overheated, the pillow too hard. It's simple, I coached myself: relax, breathe with him, and you'll fall asleep. So I modulated my breathing to be syncopated with his. But it was no use. In minutes, I'd lose track or fail to keep his rhythm. I'd lie awake, wedged between my father and the wall.

What *really* happens to a person who goes without sleep? A young doctoral student, Nathaniel Kleitman, kept himself awake for five days in the early 1920s to try to answer this question. His experiment, repeated dozens of times and involving several other subjects, was one of the first systematic studies of sleep deprivation; it became the basis of his physiology dissertation at the University of Chicago. Kleitman's research led to two intriguing conclusions. First, people who stayed up all night were actually more alert in the morning than they'd been in the middle of the sleepless night. Second, after about sixty hours of being awake, the ill effects of sleeplessness appeared to level off; health and behavior did not further degenerate even if sleep deprivation continued. Both findings invalidated the theory that fatigue-inducing toxins progressively accumulated in the body.

The hypnotoxin myth was one of many debunked by Dr. Kleitman. In an extraordinary fifty-year career, he revolutionized and modernized the study of sleep. He established the country's first sleep research laboratory, where he conducted rigorous experiments on animal and human subjects, often including himself; wrote a definitive scientific text, *Sleep and Wakefulness*, first published in 1939, which remains in print today; and in collaboration with others, made seminal discoveries about the stages of normal sleep, rapid eye movement (REM) sleep, and dreaming. Kleitman is often called, reverentially, the Dean of Sleep Research, yet the image I have of him evokes a very different title.

In an enlarged Xerox copy of a grainy 1938 newspaper photograph that hangs above my desk, he is emerging from Mammoth Cave, Kentucky, in which he and an assistant had spent thirty-two consecutive days carrying out a primitive experiment. A tall, bearded man in a black robe, Kleitman materializes from darkness, followed by a second bearded man, B. H. Richardson, in the same flowing attire. Kleitman's face is bleached as white as the druidic hood covering his head. Stunned by flashbulbs, he looks as if he's been captured against his will. He holds a kerosene lamp in his left hand.

Other details are lost to the inky blackness, yet a wild look remains in his beady eyes—the look of a man who has been to the underworld and back. It is Hypnos himself, together with Morpheus.

They lived in near total isolation from the outside world, seeking nothing less than to challenge the "cosmic forces," as Kleitman put it, that mandate the twenty-four-hour ("circadian") cycle of sleep and wakefulness. In their experiment, Kleitman and Richardson attempted to adjust to a twenty-eight-hour schedule—nineteen wakeful hours and nine in bed—a six-day week. Although food was left for them daily, and a photographer apparently visited once, "subjects R and K," as Kleitman identified his assistant and himself in scientific literature, had virtually no contact with others.

"The darkness was absolute . . . ; the silence was also complete; and the temperature was always 54 degrees Fahrenheit," Kleitman wrote of their deep cavern home, which measured sixty feet wide and twenty-five feet high. The only unpleasant factors he acknowledged were humidity that amounted to "almost complete saturation" and a family of rats. The bed legs stood in buckets of water to keep the rats away. Archival photos show scant domestic touches: a floral bedspread, pillows, a rocking chair. In one picture, R, shirtless, washes in a basin as K pours water over him; that was the extent of their bathing. The two men existed in service to their research, using lamplight to take their vital signs, record impressions, and read.

R successfully adapted to the twenty-eight-hour day, offering proof in Kleitman's mind that cosmic forces were not invincible. K's behavior was very different—he slept well only when it coincided with his usual schedule. They both quickly resumed normal twenty-four-hour sleep-wake patterns following the experiment. Kleitman later attributed K's "resistance to change" (note the hint of self-reproach) to his older age.

The resistance is older than Kleitman, as it turns out, and far older than any of us. Our bodies are little changed from prehistoric man's, scientists today believe; we share the same deeply etched biological rhythms. The impulse to awaken remains intrinsically linked to the rising of the sun. Obversely, dusk stimulates the brain's sleep mechanisms, including secretion of the hormone melatonin, which causes natural drowsiness.

Our entire lives are shaped by circadian rhythms, gravitational forces, and seasonal cycles (day and night, ebb and flow, growth and decay), all of which, in my view, may be echoed in grander schemes throughout the cosmos. None of which can truly be resisted, only tested and studied, in Kleitman's cave as in Plato's. Daylight to darkness, the body mimics the behavior of the earth itself. Perhaps this is why vexing sleep questions (Why do humans dream? Why do we wake up?) sound like great metaphysical questions about the meaning of life; excerpts from a timeless dialogue on truth and illusion, awareness and unconsciousness.

In a fantasy, I imagine Kleitman and Richardson in Mammoth Cave in the middle of the first night, pacing briskly to keep warm. "What would happen if we never fell asleep?" the younger man asks.

Kleitman extinguishes their lamp. In the perfect darkness, he responds: "What would happen if the earth never turned away from the sun?"

❧

Clearly, Kleitman had the soul of an insomniac. In him, I see a mirror image of myself: a man obsessed with sleep, who thinks about it every waking moment and views his own body as a laboratory for research. I could spend a month in a dark, quiet cave, too. It sounds like being in a perpetual state of bedtime:

shut off from the rest of the world, occupied by nothing but another man and a pile of books, and waiting for sleep to come.

It may signal its approach with a yawn, a common first sign of drowsiness. In an academic paper from the 1950s, French scientist Jacques Barbizet described the yawn as "halfway between a reflex and an expressive movement," which captures it brilliantly, linking a yawn to other spontaneous acts such as a smile or a sigh or a deeply satisfying stretch. Of course, it's not just humans who can't fight the urge—some fish yawn, for instance, as do birds, snakes, crocodiles, and closer to home, family pets. And it's been proven that, among people at least, yawning can be contagious (even reading about it can cause one). Its purpose has been plumbed over time. Some scientists believed yawning fulfilled a need to flood the blood with oxygen, while others thought it involved releasing carbon dioxide, yet both theories are incorrect. Most likely, yawning is required for periodically exercising the mouth and throat muscles—the exaggerated jaw stretch may be its only necessary element. Tiredness gives the body an excuse to yawn, as I see it, but yawning is not vital to sleep onset.

Regardless, on some nights, a good long yawn is as close as I come to a good night's sleep, so I savor each of its four to seven seconds. I picture a yawn triggering the brain to fire off a round of sleep-inducing pellets into the bloodstream; they find their targets in lolling limbs and fluttering eyelids. In the heart of a yawn is a moment of suspension—not unlike the pause immediately before orgasm—when it feels as if the yawn itself is swallowing you, an inner-ear roar rises, and all outside sound is muffled. It's a moment you'd like to go on and on, but trying to freeze a yawn is like trying to seek haven in a hiccup. And trying to re-create one is pointless—a self-induced, fake yawn is always a disappointment. If you're lucky, though, one delicious yawn is followed by another and another, and next thing you know, you're falling asleep.

Like a blown-out candle, the brain was thought for centuries to "go dark" in sleep, indistinct from its condition in other quiescent states, such as coma. Two major discoveries changed this assumption. In 1875, Scottish physiologist Richard Caton proved that the brain generates electrical activity. Fifty years later, a German psychiatrist, Hans Berger, found that this activity is measurably different when humans are awake versus asleep; he was able to detect varying rhythms through electrodes placed at the base of the head. Berger called these brain waves "electroencephalograms" or EEGs. Sleep's presence could now be captured, without ever disturbing the sleeper.

Berger's innovation marked a turning point in sleep research, providing an objective method for studying sleep and wakefulness. Subsequent scientists found that each state has a unique profile. Alert wakefulness, for example, is characterized by stormy brain activity, at a low electrical voltage and a rapid beat of up to thirty-five "beta rhythms" per second. After the eyes close for sleep, brain waves begin to slow down as the voltage gradually increases. When deep sleep settles in, the brain idles at less than four "delta rhythms" per second, picking up speed again during REM (pronounced "remm"), the stage most closely associated with dreaming. All other phases of sleep are referred to, in general, as non-REM (NREM).

EEGs can now be traced in human fetuses at as early as three months—alternating patterns of electrical activity are indistinguishable, though, so a sleep state cannot yet be defined. At this same fetal age, two of sleep's most necessary tools develop: the eyelids. One might dream up any number of lyrical analogies for the tough, supple skin that both protects the eyes and closes them, but the anatomical fact is better than anything I could ever imagine: the tissue of eyelids is most like the tissue of the scrotum. The larger upper lid is equipped with a tiny muscle, which won't fully function until the ninth month, allowing the eyes finally to open.

By seven months, scientists can detect the first true sign of sleep—fetal brain waves in alternating bursts and hesitations, two to eight seconds each. By eight months, rapid eye movements can be spotted during a sonogram, and periods of fetal activity and rest seem to be synchronous with the mother's own cycle of REM and NREM sleep. I'd like to know the exact moment when the switch is turned on and human sleep begins or, looking at it the other way, when the switch is turned off—surely, that was the instant when all of my sleep problems started. Just as sleep develops, along with organs and limbs, is there also a way in which wakefulness grows?

Perhaps driven by similar curiosity, scientists at Oxford in the early 1970s performed experiments on living, pregnant sheep and made a startling discovery: the sheep fetuses simulated breathing. Using electrophysiological measurements to "read" what was occurring in utero, the researchers detected movement in the trachea and diaphragm. Although air obviously was not filling the lungs, the scientists speculated that this breathing motion was training the respiratory system for life outside the womb. Taking that first gasp of oxygen might not be possible without it. They found that the episodes of "in utero breathing" occurred during low-voltage electrical activity, which is characteristic postnatally of both wakefulness and REM sleep. This prompted the scientists to pose a bold question: Does the fetus actually wake up while in the womb?

To answer this, researchers in the late seventies decided to look in on a fetus—literally. They implanted a clear port-hole on the belly of a pregnant sheep. With their own eyes, they were able to see a fetus nuzzling up against the window, like a manatee swimming up to a docked submarine. Strictly speaking, the sheep fetus was never awake—it did not open its eyes or move its body with the purposefulness that defines this condition. Rather, it performed gestures of wakefulness— kicking its limbs, licking its lips, sucking, swallowing, and breathing. At the same time, its brain waves clearly indicated REM sleep. Which suggests to me that it was dreaming. And while I do not have science backing me up, I'm inspired to make an even larger theoretical leap: just as in utero breathing may train the respiratory system, perhaps fetal REM sleep and dreaming train the developing brain for the demands of life after birth.

What would one dream in utero? Without visual imagery to draw upon, human fetal dreams must be composed of vastly different perceptions, more like dissonant music than a surrealist film; the sounds of maternal organs—heart, lungs, stomach—mixing with speech, laughter, crying. A dream might be choreographed from movements of the mother's body. Or maybe, just maybe, connected as it is by the umbilical cord, the baby has no dreams of its own. It dreams whatever the mother is dreaming.

My mother, Diane, an artist, was dreaming of having a boy, a desire so powerful it may have rubbed off. I was her fifth child in six years, the firstborn son. She was thirty-two at the time. My father, Patrick, was thirty-six, a West Point graduate and Korean War veteran. Their girls were ages six, four, three, and two: Colleen, Ellen, Margaret, and Shannon.

Delivered by cesarean, as was my sister before me, I can't help wondering if my parents selected my birth date deliberately, a kind of dual holy day for Irish Catholics such as us: January 6, the Feast of the Epiphany. Commonly known as the Twelfth Day of Christmas, when the three wise men finally found the manger, this day, I like to think, also observes the term *epiphany* as redefined by James Joyce: the sudden revelation, by chance word or gesture, of "whatness"—the essential nature of a thing. Eyes open or shut, my life has been a continual, awkward stumbling upon *whatnesses,* sharp fragments of unexpected meaning. It all started in 1961 at St. Barnabas Catholic Hospital in Minneapolis, around the time I like to get out of bed now, at 8:38 in the morning.

Chapter 2

≈

Lullabies

I WAS BORN dreaming. Deep in REM sleep, I was taken from the womb, my closed eyes furiously scanning for images that could never be retrieved, redreamed, or remembered. In this regard, I was identical to every baby. With a slap to the ass, it was over. Birth jolted me from a state of sublime unconsciousness to which I've spent the rest of my life struggling to return.

My eyes popped open and I let out a healthy yowl. The obstetrician, Dr. John Moehn, handed me to a nurse, who swabbed my eyelids with silver nitrate or another antibiotic to prevent infection. Air passages were cleared; fingers and toes counted; time of birth recorded. While my mother was being stitched up, someone notified my father, ready with cigars in the waiting room. I was bathed, measured, and weighed (seventeen inches; six pounds, eleven ounces). This much I know for sure. It's verified by the official record, on file with the Minnesota Department of Public Health, Section of Vital Statistics: Live Birth No. 122-61-0-00807.

It's harder to recapture authentically the sound of relief that greeted a healthy baby—and the surprise of a boy or a girl—in the days before sonograms and amniocentesis. Deliveries were secluded affairs, not the New Age family reunions arranged today, with grandparents at the stirrups, husband at bedside, and brother-in-law making a birth video. Having a baby must have seemed both more commonplace and more mysterious for women of my mother's generation and earlier.

Letters and telegrams following my birth convey these different inflections. "We really were shaky, waiting for the long-distance call yesterday," Mom's dad, Herbert, wrote to her from Denver on January 7, 1961. "Across the miles, it's a nerve-wracking experience, but not quite as tough as sitting outside the delivery-room door. *A little boy! At last!* . . . Your Dad will have you enrolled in West Point by the fall of 1981, we hope."

If my first instinct was to open my eyes, then my next instinct was to close them. I was neither attempting to return to the womb nor simply recovering from the trauma of birth. On this, I have the word of science. Like all newborns, I was more alive to the world in sleep than in wakefulness.

In our first few days of life, we commonly spend as much as eighteen of twenty-four hours asleep—more than we will ever sleep again, except during illness. Aristotle thought this was due to the infant's disproportionately large head (a trait shared with "dwarfs," he wrote, who also "are addicted to sleep"), while eighteenth-century British physician David Hartley considered it a result of the brain's "endeavour to expand itself." Hartley was close; sleep is necessary for growth.

At this age, sleep does not come in one long stretch, but in three- or four-hour cycles. It appears to be a sleep without nuance: so deep as to be nearly unarousable or so fragile as to seem irreparable. New parents often fear that their baby is deaf, for it can truly sleep through anything—blaring television or smoke detector. Then, to nothing but its own internal cues, the child suddenly wakes, wakes them up, and despite all good measures, will not fall back asleep.

The newborn behaves like an adult with severe jet lag—as frequently awake at night as asleep during the day. In fact, its condition is more extreme. Adults who arrive in a new time zone need a day or two to reset their internal clock. Newborns, fresh from nine months' darkness, require several weeks to become oriented. The baby's clock is being assembled at the same time the body first needs it. Biological rhythms begin adapting to the earth's zeitgebers, daylight and temperature, as well as to domestic cues such as feeding times and the parents' sleep schedules. By three months, though total sleep time decreases, infants stay asleep for longer stretches.

It is my unsubstantiated belief that a cure for insomnia lies somewhere in the warm, milky sleep of babies. No person fails to be tranquilized when near one. Maybe it's in their scent. Poking my head into a newborn's crib, I try to breathe it in, hoping sleep will fill my lungs—a virus that blooms every night and enfolds each morning; a quick, painless inoculation against insomnia. I'd be satisfied, I promise myself, if only I could take in a tiny bit.

I understand perfectly well what two French scientists were thinking when, in a 1907 experiment, they drew blood serum from sleepy dogs and injected it into wakeful ones. Seeing a dog napping in the middle of the day, I'm struck by a similar thought—a twist on a Joan Didion line—one I've idly considered while holding a napping baby: Give me the biochemical structure of sleep and I'll have it synthesized in a laboratory. Studying it under a microscope, I'm sure I would find an entirely different composition in newborn sleep than in my own.

Dr. Kleitman discovered as much himself. A dozen years after he staggered from Mammoth Cave, he was back in Chicago applying what he had learned underground to the sleep of babies. As a scientist and a father, Kleitman was genuinely fascinated by children (*Sleep and Wakefulness* was dedicated to daughters Hortense and Esther, both of whom were frequent research subjects, from infancy on). He believed that a baby's sleep was purest—not yet corrupted by clocks, electric light, nine-to-five, and other hindrances imposed by society.

In 1950, Dr. Kleitman began the first study of infant sleep under regular family living conditions. With the aid of some supremely cooperative parents, he tracked the behavior of nineteen infants, beginning at the third week of life and continuing for six months. Each family used a specially constructed crib that mechanically charted the baby's movements, twenty-four hours a day. (For the purpose of the study, periods of motionlessness were counted as sleep, although of course a baby can be awake yet very still.) Mothers kept careful records of the time their child spent out of the crib for feedings, diaper changes, baths, and play. The research yielded 2,873 infant days of data.

Dr. Kleitman was especially curious to learn if an infant has a "natural" daily cycle of sleep and wakefulness. Government pamphlets of the time informed parents that all babies sleep for as much as twenty-two hours. Not true, Dr. Kleitman found; sleep time ranged from twelve to seventeen hours out of twenty-four. He also determined that newborns already showed a preference to sleep more at night than by day—about two extra hours. And the trend continued. For the first fifteen weeks, the increase in night sleep almost exactly equaled the decrease in day sleep. By the sixth month, infants slept at night for ten hours and day sleep had dwindled to about three and a half hours.

One infant, Dr. Kleitman found, was an anomaly. This child's extremely indulgent parents didn't try to force regular feeding times on the newborn and let the little girl determine her own daily schedule of sleeping, waking, and eating. Like B. H. Richardson in Mammoth Cave, she established a pattern that did not conform to an "astronomically correct twenty-four hours." For the first seventeen weeks, her internal clock had an extra hour tacked on to it. If, for instance, she fell asleep at eight one night, then it was nine the next night, and ten the next, and so on. This is called *free-running*, a term that refers to a delayed circadian rhythm when zeitgebers are removed. The baby girl in Dr. Kleitman's study did finally adopt a twenty-four-hour rhythm at about five months old.

In the midst of this research, Dr. Kleitman became the faculty advisor to a University of Chicago student named Eugene Aserinsky; their meeting would ultimately have a far greater impact on our knowledge of sleep than the small-scale infant study. Aserinsky would go on to make a landmark discovery in the field: REM sleep.

⌒☙⌒

"There was no joy in this initial encounter for either of us," Dr. Aserinsky recalled in a candid article written for the *Journal of the History of Neurosciences* in 1996. He was interested in organ physiology, not sleep research—which was still "on the fringe of respectable science"—yet no other faculty member was available. "For his part, Kleitman could not have been elated with the prospect of my apprenticeship, particularly after scanning my biography, which revealed a motley background." Aserinsky, age twenty-nine, had studied Spanish language; been a dental student and a social worker; and earlier, handled high explosives while serving in the U.S. army.

Aserinsky needed to come up with a graduate school project; Kleitman mentioned a recent report he'd read in the January 1950 issue of *Nature* on the phenomenon of blinking. The author, a physicist named Robert Lawson, claimed that while riding on a passenger train he was able to pinpoint sleep onset by observing the blinking of a young married couple who dozed off several times during the trip. Blinking, Lawson wrote, stopped abruptly with sleep. Kleitman thought this was in error and that blinking, instead, stopped gradually. He instructed Aserinsky to thoroughly test the blinking hypothesis. For research subjects, he suggested that Aserinsky observe the nineteen infants currently being studied.

It was a convenient arrangement. Aserinsky was already working on the study, going home to home and providing analysis of crib readings. Plus, babies sleep during the day, which allowed the graduate student to do his work and still see his wife and son at night. It was not, however, fruitful at first. Aserinsky, who had buried himself in the literature on blinking, "thereby becoming the premiere savant in that narrow field," discovered that an infant's blink is indistinct, not comparable to the blinking of an adult. He dreaded informing his advisor. "The door between [the laboratory] and Kleitman's office engraved a permanent image upon my mind," he later recalled, "because it was opened only on relatively rare occasions and represented a sort of Berlin Wall separating two worlds. On occasion, when it was absolutely essential to communicate with Kleitman, I would knock on the door and wait for a slightly irritated, 'Yes?'"

As Aserinsky confessed to him the failure of the blinking research, "Kleitman's visage, which was always serious, now seemed gloomier. There was neither reprimand nor criticism, but I knew that silence was not an accolade." Grasping for an alternative, Aserinsky proposed studying any kind of lid movement, even one caused passively through eyeball motion. Dr. Kleitman consented and Aserinsky returned to observing the infants. After several tedious months of staring into cribs, Aserinsky began making progress. He noticed that, as soon as his little subjects fell asleep, their eyes rolled very rapidly under their lids. At first, Aserinsky misinterpreted this to be a residual waking movement and didn't think it relevant. He thought he'd made a more significant discovery in what he called the "No Eye Movement" period. In each hourly cycle of infant sleep, he'd found a twenty-minute period of complete ocular rest.

Based on the timing of the No Eye Movement period, Aserinsky was soon able to devise a formula for predicting almost the exact moment when the baby would awaken—and he could leave. "The mothers were invariably amazed at the accuracy of my prediction," he recalled, "and equally pleased by my impending departure."

Relieved as he may have been when the infant study came to an end, it also left Aserinsky without research subjects. Shifting focus, he decided to search for the adult equivalent of the No Eye Movement period he'd seen in babies. His idea was to monitor an adult's eyes throughout a whole night's sleep, something—amazingly enough—that no scientist had ever before done. In preparation, Aserinsky started to tinker with a device used for recording eye movement, an old electrooculogram (EOG) machine. A clunker that hadn't been used in years, it spontaneously spewed wild pen tracings of eye movement even when no subject was attached. Funds for a better machine weren't available, Dr. Kleitman informed Aserinsky; he'd have to make do. Since he couldn't very well try it on himself while also operating it, he enlisted his eight-year-old son, Armond, to help him calibrate the equipment.

Late in 1951, in a University of Chicago laboratory, he hooked up Armond for a nightlong test. He said good-night to his boy and settled in for the sleepless EOG vigil. To his dismay, he soon noticed that the damn machine was acting up again; though Armond was asleep, the pen tracings jerked up and down. This was just like the readings he'd gotten when his son had been awake and intentionally moving his eyes back and forth. What a disaster! Aserinsky felt sure that his research project was unraveling before him, yet as the graph paper piled up, he saw the pen tracings settle down and later shoot up again, a pattern that recurred through the night. On another evening, he repeated the test with Armond and obtained the same results.

Still unsure if his equipment was working, Aserinsky decided to use both an EOG and an EEG, which allowed him to cancel out any inaccuracies. In experiments with twenty adult subjects, he confirmed his initial findings. He was now able to tie the unusual rapid eye movements to distinct, active brain waves of about twenty minutes' duration. Following a hunch, Aserinsky conducted a second series of experiments with half the subjects; he woke them repeatedly, both in the presence and in the absence of rapid eye movement, and asked, "Did you dream? What did you see?"

Awakenings during ocular rest failed to evoke more than 17 percent dream recall, while 75 percent of those made during the eye movement period elicited detailed dreams. From this, Aserinsky speculated that he had found sleep's main dream state. Aserinsky initially thought to name it the "Jerky Eye Movement" period, but settled on the more elegant-sounding "Rapid Eye Movement" or REM sleep. With Nathaniel Kleitman, his thesis advisor, as coauthor, this series of discoveries was made public in a brief article in the journal *Science* on September 4, 1953.

Although it attracted little attention at that time, the

REM sleep discovery was historic for two reasons. It proved that sleep was not a single, unvarying state, as had been thought. It also strongly suggested that dreaming did not occur by chance, but at regular intervals. Building upon Aserinsky's primary findings, Dr. Kleitman and a new assistant, William C. Dement, verified within a few years that REM is highly correlated with dreaming, and that a predictable sequence of patterns over a night's sleep can be tracked by EEG, EOG, and other methods.

In healthy adults, sleep cycles are about ninety minutes each. A typical cycle includes five stages, the first of which is a hybrid between sleep and wakefulness and lasts only a few minutes. Stage 2, still a relatively light phase, continues for up to twenty-five minutes, evolving into a brief period of heavier sleep, stage 3. This is followed by the deepest sleep of the night, stage 4, thirty to forty minutes during which one is quite simply insensible. Abrupt body movements signal the end of stage 4 and a return to stage 1 or 2—there may even be a slight awakening—which then gives way to the fifth stage, REM. Variations on this cycle continue throughout the night, with stage 2 becoming progressively dominant toward morning, and 3 and 4 disappearing. A good night's sleep includes five cycles, each of which always ends in REM.

While adults wade through several stages before reaching REM, infants plunge right into it. Their neurological circuitry is not yet properly wired, and they're better able to process information while dreaming than while awake. Babies have just two sleep stages, split evenly: REM sleep and "Quiet Sleep," a stage in which they hardly seem to move or breathe.

In adult REM sleep, the body is in commotion. Heart rate, breathing, and blood pressure are erratic; men have erections, women have clitoral engorgement; brain waves are rapid-fire. Despite the activity, all motor muscles are paralyzed. (No wonder being chased in a dream is so terrifying: the mind is flooded with messages to run, but the legs hear nothing.) In infants, by contrast, the commands make it through because the brain mechanisms that block nerve impulses to muscles are still immature. Infants squirm and kick in REM sleep and move fingers and toes. Their faces are expressive, sometimes mimicking anger or fear. It's as if everything is being rehearsed. Babies smile for the first time while dreaming.

As effortless as it appears for most infants, sleep is an acquired skill. Mastering it depends on being well cared for—on being allowed to establish patterns that literally become imprinted on the brain. One would think that lullabies are helpful, yet they may be more soothing to adults than to babies. Some nineteenth-century scientists claimed that bedtime singing could cause irreparable harm. Writing in 1897, one expert condemned all "methods of putting children to sleep artificially . . . including monotonous and unmusical lullabies and the rocking of babies in cradles or simply in the arms." It was believed that these could cause "anemia of the brain" and "idiocy," as suggested by an old German proverb, "He has been rocked into stupidity."

If current speculation proves true, music may actually help young brains to develop—even increase intelligence, some would say—but it still doesn't promote sleep. By four months, when a baby is alert enough to notice them, lullabies are too stimulating to be sleep-inducing. Having someone sing in your ear must be like trying to sleep while a neighbor's music plays through the floorboards.

Aside from their volume, certain lullabies have a wicked tone that, to my ears, sounds menacing. A sleep-deprived parent must have written the twisted lyrics to "Rock-a-Bye, Baby." Others are striking for their desperation—more like hush-hush deals with the devil than sweet cradlesongs. In a traditional French lullaby, the frantic singer does not so much lull the baby as plead with sleep: *Come, slumber, please come!*

Slumber does not come. Come, come, slumber, come, come.
Slumber, come and embrace the child!

❧

Some people have a constitution for yowling babies, a *way* with them. I do not. Never mind that I grew up in a virtual sorority, wherein each of my sisters, once old enough, baby-sat neighborhood kids. This seemed like easy money to me—fifty cents an hour to play games and watch TV—but baby-sitting was strictly a girl's vocation. As a boy, I had to walk dogs, wash cars, water lawns for neighbors on vacation, and shovel snow. Although I pride myself now on having a highly developed maternal instinct, my specialty is attending to the childlike needs of adults. The fierce composure needed for quieting actual infants has never been part of my package.

Twelve years ago, two of my sisters visited from Seattle with their new sons: Sam, one and a half years old, and Dylan, eight months. My sisters and their husbands got together with another young couple, who lived here in San Francisco and had a six-month-old named Megan. While they all went out for dinner, my boyfriend of the time, Nick, and I stayed home to baby-sit. We were qualified in only the vaguest of all possible ways: I was related by blood; and Nick, at thirty-seven, was several years older than any of us. The babies were the only ones not fooled.

We were left in charge of six bottles of breast milk and three wriggling bundles, as cute as lambs. I think a whole hour passed without incident. I was playing with Sam and Megan when Nick put Dylan into a high chair to feed him a bottle. For himself, he opened a nice merlot. Sipping a little wine, he blithely shared an appetizer with Dylan: ripe figs and a chunk of Gorgonzola. That cheese had more blue veins than a junkie's arm.

At first, the baby seemed fine. Then, right about the time the Gorgonzola dropped into Dylan's small intestine, mingling with figs and mother's milk, his crying started. He was not a happy child. I must say, in retrospect, it wasn't the crying itself that was so unnerving, nor that the other two babies joined in, nor that for two hours the three would not stop. No, what I still recall—indeed, can still hear—is how bloody loud it was. They cried louder than I could attempt to cry now, no matter how sick or aggrieved I might be, which is what seemed so unnatural. They had turned into ferocious little calves, bawling and bucking in our arms, thrusting their fat limbs, as if being taken for slaughter. We'd become the novice stableboys; they could no doubt smell our fear.

Operating on the theory that the crying was contagious, we separated the three: Nick rocked Dylan in one room, I wrangled Sam in another, we stuck Megan in a stroller in the hallway. With no traditional French lullabies in his repertory, Nick crooned along to a record on the stereo: Chaka Khan singing "Sweet Thing." The effect was negligible, as far as I could hear. I would have played a much darker tune: Rickie Lee Jones, practically nodding out in midsong, slurring "Coolsville."

Long past bedtimes, the babies cried even louder, their terror exceeded only by our own. We tried bottles, changed diapers; nothing worked. Picking up the phone, I tracked down my sisters at the restaurant. Dylan's mom instructed me to wrap him up and take him for a walk—a remedy meant as much for me, I was to learn later, as for the baby. Almost as soon as we went outdoors, the unmistakable scent of fresh baby's poop cut the cool night air. Relieved at last, Dylan stopped crying, which in baby code evidently meant Sam and Megan could, too. By the time their mothers finally arrived, all three babies were asleep and the bottle of merlot was empty.

I don't know how my own mother kept her wits: she had

twice as many babies within nine years. And she says she'd have loved to have had six more. Mom did have help for a time; a college student named Mary Ann lived with our family as a nanny for about four years after I was born. Yet one extra pair of arms could not always have been enough. There must have been times when half of us were in some stage of sleep while the others were in some cranky stage of wakefulness—what Mom would probably have identified as Hungry, Wet, Naughty, or Tired. Sleep scientists have come up with their own four categories, though not nearly as descriptive: Alert, Nonalert, Fuss, and Cry. I'd add an even more troublesome one, Colic, whose behavior is so extreme and widespread it could be considered a fifth state of infant wakefulness.

Colic causes one-fourth of all babies to cry for hours, for no apparent reason, usually at the exact same time in the evening, week after week. It simultaneously drives some sleep-deprived parents to their own paroxysms of crying. Others take it out on babies in ghastly acts of abuse—shaking the infants or suffocating them with a hand over the mouth. In fact, recent research has uncovered that some deaths attributed to sudden infant death syndrome (SIDS) were actually cases of infanticide.

Conventional wisdom says that colic is a sign of abdominal pain caused by gas, but antacids and similar drugs rarely stop the crying. Antispasmodics and mild tranquilizers have also been tried, to no avail. Colic is untreatable for the simple fact that there is no illness to treat. A colicky baby is, by definition, inconsolable. In controlled research studies, comparing the soothed with the unsoothed, scientists have found that nearly all colicky babies do not respond to rhythmic rocking, carrying, singing, suckling, or other measures. Which is not to say such babies should not be held or sung lullabies. Yet parents should not expect the crying to cease. As one specialist points out, saying a baby "has colic" is like saying a teenager "has adolescence." It is a natural stage of human development.

Just as a single crying spell can suddenly end—all at once, for instance, the baby falls asleep—colic stops cold by the fourth month. Even in premature infants, colic ends within four months after the original, full-term due date. This phenomenon is recognized throughout the world. The Chinese have a good phrase for it: colic is called "one hundred days of crying," as if it were a spiritual journey. It is right around this one hundredth day of life, interestingly, that alternating sleep and wake states fall into place: circadian rhythms are in sync with daylight, and the brain is regularly secreting melatonin at nighttime.

This intersection of developments has inspired a new theory: a colicky baby may be having more difficulty than others making the transition from wakefulness to sleep. At the end of the day, it finds itself stuck in a painful state of being, a nightmare of consciousness, no more able to fall asleep than someone in a coma is to awaken. Trapped, the baby cries and cries, until it finally cries itself to sleep.

I cried so much in my first weeks that my parents thought I had colic. I'd like to think it was really a neonatal existential crisis, but all signs point to something less melodramatic and more fixable. Born into an Irish family that owned a small ice cream company (Minneapolis's Jersey Ice Cream, founded in 1890 by my dad's grandfather, after whom I was named), I was allergic to the very thing upon which our livelihood depended: cow's milk. In my imagination, whenever my mother (pregnant with me) ate that rich ice cream—higher in butterfat, the family legend goes, than any other brand before or since—it made its way into my bloodstream and into my fetal dreams. By birth, I'd had my fill. My parents obviously didn't know I was allergic—they bottle-fed me milk, breast-feeding being both out of fashion in 1961 and impractical for a mother with four toddlers. But they figured it out soon enough. I expressed my discontent with the world in the only way I knew how: through sleep—or rather, through the lack thereof.

Of course, I remember none of this. Infants have no memories. It may be more correct to say, we retain no memories of infancy. There's no way for the brain to store them. Only as the baby's brain matures does the capacity to remember develop. The absence of early memories has a lovely parallel in how the brain functions at the onset of sleep. Shortly after the eyelids close, the link between short- and long-term memory shuts down. If something doesn't make it into long-term storage by roughly three minutes before falling asleep, the memory is lost. Likewise, if sleep goes uninterrupted, we cannot remember dreams that occur through the night, only those just prior to wakening.

Our first years of life are like those last three minutes before sleep: a synaptic gap of nothing but drowsiness. If we have impressions, most likely we've assumed them from someone else. Perhaps we've picked up the family story, rethreaded a hundred times through the eye of a dull needle.

I was "a good baby," my parents invariably recall, and I "slept well"—once they switched me to formula. A saved lock of hair shows that I was blond. Other features are recognizable from snapshots, tinted as if with colored chalk. In one, I'm surrounded by sisters, cousins, and grandparents and am dressed in a light-blue military suit with gold braided epaulets and a matching cap.

Within two years of my birth, Mom was pregnant again. My sister Julia was born in October 1963, a few months after my dad's mother died of Lou Gehrig's disease. His father had passed away shortly before—at a Sunday supper, his head had dropped onto his chest and he was gone, Dad has said, as though he'd just turned out the lights. A formidable pair, Lil and Frank were an authentic mom-and-pop, and their deaths left the ice cream company at loose ends. Dad sold his inherited shares to his younger brother, avoiding an inevitable feud between them over joint ownership. Even knowing that history, I have a hard time understanding why my father—eldest son and first in line—left a third-generation family business with a seemingly prosperous future. As it turned out, he made a smart move. Within a year, every last pint of hand-packed Jersey Ice Cream would be gone; the manufacturing plant and surrounding area were razed to make room for a freeway.

What was my father thinking at the time? When asked, he remembers one thing: he needed to find a way to support his family. It seems to me he was dreaming. At thirty-eight, he bought a Coca-Cola bottling plant in Spokane, a town he had visited just once before, twelve hundred miles away. The son of an ice cream man would go West, with wife and kids, to become a purveyor of caffeinated soda.

⤖

Chapter 3

Dream of Flying

I CAN SEE the family moving from our Minneapolis home. The memory is fixed by photography. Black-and-white snapshots, fingered like old playing cards, both trace and distort our steps. I don't honestly recall our having lived in the crisp white house on Abbott Place, yet I recognize it from the outside by its boxy, dark window shutters and square, birthday-present shape. Inside, I know there is a winding gray staircase leading to a second floor; I am pictured on it, age three, seated next to my sister Shannon, who's five. She holds a favorite doll, likely pulled from the moving box behind us. We wear boots and dark winter coats, dressed to go. It is 1964, the middle of January.

In Mom's home movies taken at the Minneapolis airport,

I am held by Mary Ann, who moved with us, as my older sisters wave to the camera before boarding the aircraft. They are energetically waving back at themselves, it seems to me now, saying hello again and again, not good-bye. My father isn't in these pictures; he had moved out to Spokane two months earlier to take over the Coke bottling plant. The movie continues on the plane, where I sit in Mary Ann's lap before takeoff, drowsy-eyed, looking like a shutdown ventriloquist's dummy.

The film stops there and the familiar details burn off to bare a memory that could not be handed down or photographed: the sensation of flying. I have no sense of time, of going from here to there, or of traveling to rejoin my father, but a hazy perception of being up high, snow-fringed ground replaced by sky, winter cold by cabin heat, and ferocious engines by a deep, sleep-inducing hum.

Perhaps I nodded off and what I recollect is a childhood dream, one that is common to humans of every age, a dream of flying. Like their converse, dreams of falling, flying dreams often take place in the drowsy passage between wakefulness and sleep, termed the *hypnagogic state* by French scientist Alfred Maury in the 1840s. (It is pronounced "hip-nuh-goj-ik.") Although dream*like*, the sensations of "falling asleep" are closer to hallucinations and may be equally pleasant or terrifying. They occur while the brain is technically in a waking state and lack the complex narrative thread of REM stage dreams. Often lasting only seconds and characterized by feelings of weightlessness, these experiences frequently end with a jerk, as if one had suddenly crashed to the ground, heart pounding. A physiological response to a chimerical scene, "hypnic jerks" are likely caused by misfired messages from the brain as muscles prepare to sleep.

Particularly in the late nineteenth century, physicians and neurologists avidly studied the hypnagogic state, Freud among them; it was thought to be a medium for the unguarded *self*, not subject to the waking will. Certain that the hypnagogic state would reveal the mind's deeply buried ills, exposing sources of hysteria and neuroses, they were fascinated by its similarities to hypnotic trance, fainting spells, sleepwalking, and other peculiar states of "feeble pathological consciousness," as Russian scientist Marie de Manacéine wrote in her 1897 book, *Sleep: Its Physiology, Pathology, Hygiene, and Psychology*. She tartly advised that hypnagogia is "not of good augury."

De Manacéine, a prolific writer and one of the first female physicians in Russia, had a flare for dramatic pronouncements. "Ennui," she wrote, "must induce sleep," a line that I've become fond of reciting at bedtime. Purely by the sound of her writing voice—astringent yet sensual—I imagine de Manacéine to be a brilliant elderly oddball; Marie Curie meets Julia Child, with the bemused face of Colette. She wrote of sleep lovingly, as a mysterious anthropomorphic entity, and at times approached her subject with a fierce protectiveness: "It would be difficult to find any aspect of life towards which so much injustice and ingratitude have been shown as towards sleep," she stated in the book's opening pages. In another passage, it was as if she were writing metaphorically about creatures like herself: "Men are only interested in sleep so far as it satisfies their love of the marvellous."

Prominent in the Victorian era of sleep research, de Manacéine is known today for having performed the first studies of sleep deprivation in animals. In 1894, she proved that puppies died when kept awake for up to six days, an experiment that tarnishes my image of her. I picture Madame de Manacéine, like Madame Defarge, knitting through the night in her laboratory while she mercilessly watched their heads fall.

More than a third of de Manacéine's book was devoted to dreaming, with a long section on hypnagogia. She felt sure that this "half-waking state" was an early symptom of insanity.

In another claim that has since been disproved, de Manacéine stated that dreams of flying and falling are most common in very young children. She thought this might be because children sleep so intensely and have "ample occasions to familiarize themselves with the sensations of falls."

An omnivorous theorist, de Manacéine cited the ideas of Kant, Voltaire, and Goethe, as well as colleagues such as William Alexander Hammond, an American physician who was of the singular opinion that hypnagogic hallucinations were induced by a glass of champagne or "a few drops of laudanum," the chief ingredient of which is opium. In a footnote, de Manacéine also referenced G. Stanley Hall, editor of *The American Journal of Psychology*. Dr. Hall (as much transcendentalist poet as psychologist, it seems) felt that dreams of flying offered "some faint reminiscent atavistic echo from the primeval sea." Our ancestors "were not birds, and we cannot inherit sensations of flying," he pointed out, "but they floated and swam for longer than they have had legs. Why may there not be vestigial traces of this in the soul?" Reflecting upon himself, Hall wrote that "sensations of hovering, gliding by an inner impulse rather than by limbs, falling and rising, have been from boyhood very real both sleeping and waking."

His science may be dubious, but I admire his gift for reminiscence. If I am to recall my entire life, I also wish to reach as far back in time as possible. I'd like to think that, as the plane was lifting off from Minneapolis, I was hearing strains of a faint "atavistic echo"; not falling asleep, but rather in the earliest stage of waking. The scientific term for this state is *hypnopompic,* combining *Hypnos* with the Greek word *pompe,* literally "sending sleep away."

Thinking about that morning now, I remember looking down through the small plane window. I can make out the neatly quilted ground and the clouds swirling, as though I were watching bedclothes in a slow, slow washing machine.

But I may very well have superimposed them, a few hypnopompic props and some color added in or taken from a later plane trip. It is sun through the window and the aircraft's hum that I recall most vividly—heat on my face and a soft purring I could feel through the seat. I must have pulled away from Mary Ann or my mother, pressed my face against the window, or placed my chin on the sill. Like an alarm, the engine rumble took root, causing teeth to ring, skull to buzz. This is how I first remember myself, the moment I came into consciousness.

Preposterous, Nathaniel Kleitman would no doubt say, if he were here to challenge me. I mean here in my apartment. Perhaps his office would be more suitable. Indeed, I've attempted to make an appointment with the great sleep doctor.

Since first encountering his work, I presumed him dead. He was born in Kishinev, Russia, in 1895, before my own grandparents, all of whom passed away long ago. While searching for his obituary, however, I discovered to my complete astonishment that, 104 years later, Nathaniel Kleitman was still alive. "Alive and kicking," as one of his professional associates described him. He was living proof of his own sleep deprivation experiments: insomnia has no adverse effect on human life span. I learned that Dr. Kleitman resided in southern California, cared for by his daughter Esther. My request for an interview was cordially yet unequivocally denied. Esther Kleitman, who is nearly my mother's age, sent regrets on her father's behalf, without explanation.

I do not need him in the flesh, though. Dr. Kleitman's thoughts and findings are encapsulated in his 550-page opus, *Sleep and Wakefulness.* First published in 1939 and substantially revised for a 1963 edition, the book's most important legacy for researchers today may be its bibliography of sleep-related literature; it lists 4,300 sources spanning two thousand years, from the classical to the modern age, in ten languages.

Paging through the bibliography provides the kind of idle pleasure one used to find at a library by randomly pulling a drawer in an old-fashioned card catalog—obscure titles piquing interest as you flipped through it. "Laughter in Dreams," a 1945 article, for example, caught my eye one day, setting me off in search of the original at a medical library and then leading me to other works by its author, Martin Grotjahn.

Grotjahn, a German immigrant, lived in Chicago at the same time as Nathaniel Kleitman. I suspect they knew one another, though they had little in common professionally: Grotjahn was a Freudian psychoanalyst, a specialty that Dr. Kleitman disdained. (Freud himself received a single, brief reference in *Sleep and Wakefulness*.) In any event, Kleitman did seem to admire certain aspects of Grotjahn's work, such as his rigorous phenomenological study of awakening. In a cited 1942 article in *The Psychoanalytic Review*, Grotjahn recorded every characteristic of the process, even categorizing types of awakening—The Slow Awakening, Awakening At An Intended Time, etc.—as if observing subtle behavioral differences in identical white lab mice.

"On special occasions," he wrote, for instance, "awakening people report that they address themselves as though they were bossing themselves with a short command 'to get up.' " This was typical of Awakening Daily At The Same Time. "They act like people who write themselves postcards so as not to forget something that they planned to do." With regard to Sudden Spontaneous Awakening, Grotjahn noted, "It is by no means self-evident that the person knows at the moment of awakening *who* he is any more than that he always knows *where* he is."

First published in German in 1932, Grotjahn's study was meant to provide insight into daily "Ego disintegration and Ego reconstruction," as exemplified in sleeping, dreaming, and awakening. "Awakening is completed when the Ego synthesis is performed," he wrote in his conclusion. Such lines sound comical today, like a snatch of dialogue from a wonderfully bad sci-fi movie. On first reading, I couldn't imagine why Kleitman, a physiologist, would even have taken notice of Grotjahn's findings. But now I suspect he overlooked the Freudian gobbledygook. At the heart of their work, both men shared an intense interest in the waking state; it was, in fact, the subject that first drew Kleitman to the field of sleep. Beyond the scientific challenges it presented, he never fully elucidated why the waking state had so captured his attention. There might be a clue in his own character. In contrast to sleeping or dreaming, to be awake is to be grounded in reality—a preferable state, I'd think, for someone as rational and disciplined as Nathaniel Kleitman.

At age seventeen, he emigrated to Palestine to attend medical school and three years later, as a war refugee in 1915, arrived at Ellis Island. While working nights in a New York pastry shop, Kleitman earned a bachelor's degree from what is now City College and a master's in science from Columbia. For two years, he was an instructor at the University of Georgia. After receiving his Ph.D. at the University of Chicago in 1923, he was awarded a fellowship to study in Paris with the psychologist Henri Piéron, one of the world's leading authorities on sleep. In 1925, Kleitman became a faculty member at the University of Chicago, where he taught without a break for the next thirty-five years before being forced to retire at age sixty-five.

Unlike scientists before him, he did not see sleep and wakefulness as opposites, but as alternating phases of the same cycle, "the one completing the other as the trough of a wave completes its crest." In Kleitman's theory, first proposed in his book's 1939 edition, sleep arrives inevitably and gracefully when stimulation diminishes to the brain's "wakefulness center." In short, "Without wakefulness, sleep cannot be said to exist."

His interest in the subject extended, tellingly, to finding the perfect word in English. "The word *sleep* is short and its meaning in everyday discourse unambiguous, but there is no satisfactory word in English for denoting the state of being awake," Dr. Kleitman observed in the *Sleep and Wakefulness* introduction. "Vigilance, and adjectives suffixed by *ness*— alertness, attentiveness, watchfulness, sleeplessness—have been equated with wakefulness and often used to indicate a state of being 'wide-awake.' *Wake* is short, but has several specialized meanings unrelated to sleep. The coined term *awakeness* has been proposed but not generally accepted. I shall, therefore, use *wakefulness*, long and awkward as it may be." At least in English, he later admitted, the term was easier to pronounce than in Russian.

Wakefulness is often incorrectly used as a synonym for *consciousness*, he pointed out. The latter does not depend upon the former. Nor—to correct another misconception—is sleep an unconscious state. It is distinct from coma, anesthesia, and a drunken stupor, Dr. Kleitman noted. Sleep, in fact, is partly characterized by the ability to awaken oneself.

"If sleep and wakefulness may be crudely likened to the dichotomy of solid ice and liquid water, which can be distinguished from each other by mere inspection, levels of consciousness are analogous to the degrees on a thermometer scale. There is only one dimension of consciousness running through sleep and wakefulness." However, the "level" of consciousness does fluctuate; "it is determined by the degree of one's ability to utilize the past and contribute to the future." In essence, therefore, consciousness is defined by two criteria: the ability to remember and to process experience.

Would my boyhood memory of flying have met Dr. Kleitman's criteria? I was alert to noise, heat, the sky, as if my senses were turned on at high volume; I was aware of myself as separate from my mother, separate from the aircraft. Still, I know this wouldn't be enough for him. It's far too subjective. In the same way that it's difficult to determine the exact instant a person wakes up, Dr. Kleitman felt that the transition from "the primitive nonconscious wakefulness" of a newborn to full consciousness does not occur all at once.

If I were to meet with him, he would demand of me unassailable proof, exactly as he had of Eugene Aserinsky when the student came to him in 1951, claiming to have discovered the existence of REM. He presented numerous polygraphic recordings of subjects in REM sleep, including his son. As Dr. Aserinsky later wrote, the evidence seemed irrefutable. But Dr. Kleitman wanted to see the "wiggling" eyes for himself. He gave Aserinsky a small home-movie camera.

Mindful of the blinding floodlights required for filming, Aserinsky rigged up a dimmer switch to raise their brightness gradually while his sleeping subjects progressed toward REM. To enhance visibility, their eyelids had been blackened with greasepaint. The camera was held close to the subjects' faces and made a loud whirring noise, Aserinsky later recalled; he was sure they'd wake up. They didn't. Hence, by accident, he'd found that in REM, a sleeper's resistance to arousal was quite high, a previously unknown aspect of this state. Because of its distinctive EEG, he had thought of it before as a variant of wakefulness.

Aserinsky returned to Dr. Kleitman's office to show his "home movies." But even this documentation was not enough. The doctor would not be convinced until he had observed a session in the sleep laboratory. For a subject, Dr. Kleitman insisted upon using one of his daughters. Finally he was satisfied. The data confirmed that REM sleep occurred with tremendous activation of the brain—a finding in direct con-

flict with his own earlier "wave" theory, a basis of Dr. Kleitman's international renown, which held that sleep was essen-
tially a passive process. Once the results were published, according to Aserinsky, Dr. Kleitman tried to take primary credit
for the discovery. Allegedly, he also refused to approve granting
Aserinsky his doctorate degree, saying that his work had been
insufficient.

What is one to make of this? Am I to admire the older
scientist for his demanding, meticulous ways or find his behavior, if true, to be petty, shameful? For his part, Aserinsky
felt that Kleitman acted "in a manner that was uncon-
scionable," like someone bitterly defending his reputation.
The work did take place in the senior doctor's laboratory,
nonetheless; it had been done on assignment. Maybe, then, it
was the younger man who had been disrespectful of his elder.

Dr. Kleitman had little to say on the matter. *Sleep and
Wakefulness* does not contain a word about Aserinsky, except
in the bibliography. As coauthor of the now legendary 1953
Science article announcing the discovery of REM, the name
E. Aserinsky is listed before the name N. Kleitman.

Chapter 4

~

Caffeinism

MY INSOMNIAC fate was sealed when the plane touched down in Spokane. Dad ran the city's main pop factory from the time I was a little boy until the year I left for college. I drank so much Coca-Cola growing up, I cannot take a sip of it today. I've often wondered if all that sugar and caffeine altered my neurochemical makeup, turning me into the alert, anxious man I am. I suspect it still runs in my veins at night, nourishing sleeplessness. My wild speculations remain unproven, however. The half-life of caffeine in adults is four to six hours, not thirty-six years.

My Coca-Cola childhood was privileged, when I think about it now. As the milkman delivered milk in the morning, so Dad brought home pop at night. But there was more to it than an endless supply of soft drinks. Once or twice a season, for example, we got to drive to church in a bright red, flatbed Coke truck. These occasions seemed a fun improvisation by my father; in reality, they probably meant that both our cars were dead. Smitty, the bottling-plant mechanic, would drop off a spare truck early Sunday morning. He wore cowboy boots and a grease-stained Coke uniform. A fidgety, silent man, always smoking, he rode in the front seat, to be driven back to the plant on the way to St. Augustine's. Mom stayed home with the baby. My older sisters and I perched atop empty yellow Coke cases in the back of the flatbed, imperial on makeshift thrones. Waving to neighbor kids, loving every bump, we felt incredibly lucky, as if we'd been chosen to ride on a parade float.

I can still see my father through the cabin window, working the pedals and the gear shift. He's dressed for church as he would be for work: a pale blue seersucker suit; white, button-down shirt; and necktie with military insignia. At age five, I, too, am in suit and tie. My sisters—seven to twelve—wear dresses and gloves; mantillas and bobby pins are entangled in their hair. Laughing, we hold on to the sides of the truck as Dad veers into the church lot, clipping the garden wall. Father Austen comes outside at that very moment, assembling his altar boys for the processional. Under the old priest's doubtful gaze, and following a couple botched runs, Dad finally parallel parks the unwieldy vehicle.

Aside from occasionally driving a Coke truck to church, our family blended right in to Spokane, a town of 180,000 in the early 1960s. It was known as the Hub of the Inland Empire, the largest city in an area comprising western Montana, northern Idaho and Oregon, and eastern Washington. The region's original inhabitants had been the Spokane Indians; like the nearby Coeur d'Alene, Walla Walla, and other tribes, they'd been moved to reservations and were almost never seen in town. The Spokane Indians baseball team did not, in fact, include any Spokane Indians. Everyone living around us was also from the Midwest, white, and Roman Catholic, with one partial exception: my mother. Mom, whom Dad teasingly called a "heathen," had not yet converted from Protestantism. Their "mixed marriage" wasn't further discussed. A family of eight such as ours was not unusual. In St. Augustine parish, one drew suspicion in two main ways: by being childless or by being conspicuously fertile (which is to say, sexual), like the Vandervoorts, whose sixteen kids spilled into two pews.

We lived on the South Hill, "the good part of town," a neighborhood of newly built homes and young middle-class families. The typical house was one-story, ranch style, with four to five bedrooms, and large front and back lawns. For several years, our house, three-quarters of the way down the street, was the last one built on Comstock Court, as if progress needed a good breather before resuming. Unlike the neighborhood's other houses, ours had a round kitchen window facing the street; it framed my mother's face when she worked over the sink. Inside, we had fine wood floors and three fireplaces, each made from a different kind of stone, and most extravagant of all, five bathrooms. Behind us, an unfenced yard gave way to several acres of wooded land—a forest of gnomes and faeries, from a child's perspective. Beyond the vacant lots to the west were paths to a bluff where we could watch the trains roll into Spokane.

The east end of Comstock Court opened onto a giant public park with swing sets, horseshoe pits, swimming pools, a baseball field, a towering flagpole at its center, and a school. My older sisters were enrolled at the tiny Comstock Elementary (one room for each grade, first through sixth), located no more than a hundred yards from our front door. The family doctor (my best friend's dad) lived within a few blocks, as did a dentist, orthodontist, dermatologist, and cardiologist. A fire station was around the corner, a bomb shelter in a house up the street. It was like growing up on the grounds of a sprawling Anglo-Saxon estate, protected from the outside world.

On our block, nothing made an impression quite like having a huge, twenty-five-foot Coke truck parked in the driveway. It meant that one of Dad's men was making a special delivery; my parents were probably having a cocktail party that night. Just sitting there—stop-sign red, daring to be trespassed—the truck drew kids on a hot summer day quicker than the sound of firecrackers. With the side panel slid open, it was like coming upon a treasure chest: stacked in pallets, row upon row of pop bottles in different flavors, as bright as gemstones.

To the other kids, it must have seemed as if a fountain of free soda fizzed and gurgled behind our front door. Which was not far from the truth. No other family had a separate refrigerator in the basement, as we did, filled with Coke and the other pops my father sold: Dad's Root Beer, Sprite, Orange Fanta, Grape and Strawberry Crush, as well as the adult flavors, Tab, Schweppes Bitter Lemon, Ginger Ale, and Fresca. If the chilled supply was low, warm cases were always stacked nearby. Like a feeder hooked up for lab animals, the Coke cooler was never empty. Thirsty, hot, bored, tired, we helped ourselves to its bottles of cold, bubbly sugar water. Day and night, the fridge hummed benevolently.

There were some limits to our consumption. No pop for breakfast, as I recall, although it was permitted while watching Saturday-morning cartoons. No more if you spilled one (an accident more likely to occur in Dad's presence). It seems to me there were further rules placed on Grape Crush and the other colorful drinks that dyed your tongue (and Mom's furniture) purple, orange, or pink. They had no value whatsoever, except for tasting good. Coca-Cola, by contrast, had a long history as a curative.

When Coca-Cola syrup was introduced in 1886, it was a "patent medicine," sold by druggists. In his text for the bottle label, the inventor John Pemberton claimed, "This Intellectual Beverage and Temperance Drink contains the valuable Tonic and Nerve Stimulant properties of the Coca plant and Cola (or Kola) nuts, and makes not only a delicious, exhilarating, refreshing and invigorating Beverage (dispensed from the soda water fountain or in other carbonated beverages), but a valuable Brain Tonic and a cure for all nervous affections—Sick Head-Ache, Neuralgia, Hysteria, Melancholy, etc." The only problem it could not solve, apparently, was sleeplessness.

Pemberton's original secret formula contained a jolting mixture of caffeine and cocaine—delightfully effective, I'm sure, after several glasses at the soda fountain. Too many, though, and it was habit-forming. Indeed, a slang term arose for people addicted to it, *Coca-Cola Fiends,* a turn-of-the-century version of *coke fiends.* Cocaine had long since been removed from Coca-Cola when I was a boy, and its primary health claims disproved, but the beverage was still considered medicinal. Coke was good for you in some unnameable way. In our home, it was routinely prescribed for headaches and diarrhea. Coca-Cola was the antidote to stomach flu, the only good thing about throwing up. At such times, Mom served it in a glass with a paper straw, along with a plate of Ritz crackers.

It is no great surprise that a household centered around Coca-Cola would have a dependent child or two. I was particularly fond of it. Although I don't drink it nowadays, I still have great affection for the classic Coke bottle. Perfectly designed eighty years ago, its hobble-skirt shape concealed nothing. Made of limpid, watery-green glass, it existed to be held, to be seen, and to be seen through. Even when warm, the bottle looked cold, as if carved from ice. And the bottle fit so nicely in the hand; one gripped it like another hand. Perhaps that was an aspect of Coca-Cola I found comforting as a child. Unquestionably, though, my attachment depended most upon the factory where it was bottled; upon the idea that it was *home*made in an essential way, a product of my father's.

Then, as now, a twelve-ounce bottle contained thirty-six milligrams of caffeine, about one-third the amount in a strong cup of coffee, the deleterious effects of which range from mild jitteriness to heart palpitations. (Until 1983, there was no such thing as caffeine-free Coke.) Some days I drank so much of it, I was, for lack of a better phrase, drunk on the stuff. Borrowing Pemberton's word, it soothed my "affections." It also inflamed them: a nervous boy, I was made more nervous by Coca-Cola.

Caffeine is a naturally occurring stimulant, a methylxanthine, which increases blood pressure and acts principally on the central nervous system. It has a potent effect on mood, recent research confirms. Many individuals report an elevated feeling of alertness on caffeine; in others, an increase in anxiety. Some researchers claim that it can cause cancer and other life-threatening illnesses; in women, it may contribute to miscarriage and osteoporosis. However, for nearly every accusation leveled against caffeine, there's a report to debunk it. Other studies show caffeine in a good light—Parkinson's disease in men, for instance, may be prevented by high caffeine intake. The drug can be found in surprising amounts in certain headache remedies, diet pills, sports drinks, and bittersweet chocolate. A few noncola soft drinks, such as Mountain Dew and Sunkist Orange, actually have more caffeine than Coca-Cola. There's now caffeinated bottled water, chewing gum, and lipstick. Can a transdermal patch be far off?

In his 1869 treatise *Sleep and Its Derangements*, William

Alexander Hammond provided an early view of the effects of caffeinated drinks: "In persons of fair and thin skins, who are not accustomed to the use of these beverages, the face can be seen to flush after they have been taken; and I have frequently met with persons in whom their use was always followed by a suffusion of the eyes, and a feeling of fullness within the head. Their power to increase the force and brilliancy of our thoughts, and to sustain the mind under depressing influences, has long been recognized."

Hoping to confirm such assumptions about caffeine's benefits, the Coca-Cola Company in 1911 commissioned a psychology professor at Barnard College, H. L. Hollingworth, to conduct a series of rigorous experiments. Dr. Hollingworth, author of *The Oblivescence of the Disagreeable* and *The Psychology of Drowsiness*, among other little-known texts, recruited sixteen students, teachers, and housewives, ages nineteen to thirty-nine, for a brutal caffeine boot camp. Divided into four "squads," each receiving either a daily placebo or caffeine capsule in a variety of doses (without knowing which), they were tested at least five times a day for forty consecutive days in tedious motor skills and mental tasks. In one test, they had to tap a metal rod four hundred times as rapidly as possible on a small metal base. Another measured the steadiness of an outstretched arm while holding a long pole. For a typing test, subjects had to type the same three-page essay, British scholar John Ruskin's "Sesame and Lilies," seven times daily. There were also memory tests, math calculations, and on and on.

"The interpretation is obscure but the facts are plain," Dr. Hollingworth stated in the concluding remarks to his study: moderate daily consumption of caffeine increased one's "capacity for work" and generally improved performance, though exactly how the drug operated within the body, he added, remained a mystery. More revealing than his comments were those collected from the study participants. Each person kept a daily journal, and after the study ended, their entries were matched to how much caffeine they had consumed.

"Brain unusually active, so much so that it gave me a wild kind of feeling and I did not like to stay alone," a thirty-three-year-old female member of Squad IV, Subject #5, reported on March 1, 1911. What #5 did not know was that she had earlier consumed six grains of caffeine—the highest dose administered—roughly equivalent to gulping down four cups of coffee in one sitting.

On caffeine days, Hollingworth noticed, the journal entries were always longer and in greater detail. Subject #11, also a female member of Squad IV, felt "dizzy and stupid" after being given four grains of caffeine on February 24. "Had no ambition to move or think till about 2:00," she wrote, following which this twenty-seven-year-old housewife charted a day of manic, slightly paranoid behavior. "Gradual rise of spirits till 4:00, then a period of exuberance, of good feeling. Fanciful ideas rampant. Had three sudden attacks of perspiration. Gradual decrease of exhilaration but continued sensations such as felt after shock. Trembling of knees and hands. Uncertainty as to truth of ideas, so feel cautious."

Most participants in the Hollingworth study reported sleeping worse than usual after consuming caffeine—"just a few winks" some nights, or none at all. In human studies conducted in the 1930s, Dr. Kleitman confirmed that large amounts of caffeine cause disturbed sleep in people of every age, a conclusion that has since been reiterated many times. Specifically, caffeine can reduce total sleep time as well as the deep, restful sleep of stages 3 and 4. Put another way, it increases wakefulness. This may explain why one of my sharpest memories from nursery school is nap time. What a strange ritual! One moment we're scribbling with crayons, the next, the drapes are ominously being closed. Mrs. Smith, in high heels, is tiptoeing around the room, shushing, and pushing down recalcitrant heads. Lying on my mat on the blue-and-white linoleum, I'd see other kids nod off, then wait for the eclipse to pass and snack time to begin.

Is it possible that caffeine somehow remained in my system? Maybe I was just uncomfortable sleeping on the floor among twenty-five squirmy bodies. Maybe we were all just pretending. Regardless, I seem to have passed the test without learning anything. On my Westminster Day School report card, I received the highest grade in "Rest Time." (What would have been criteria for failure?—*steals covers, wets mat, does not use a quiet voice while sleeptalking?*)

Caffeine is certainly unique in one way: it's the only psychoactive drug that can legally be purchased by children. But what happens when a kid with a caffeine habit goes cold turkey? While caffeine withdrawal is well understood in adults, only in the last few years have scientists studied it in kids. For a 1998 study, researchers at the University of Minnesota Medical School recruited thirty schoolchildren, ages eight to twelve, who already drank caffeinated soda regularly. The children were given about three cans of caffeinated soda daily for thirteen days followed by caffeine-free soda for one day. Then they were tested for classic withdrawal symptoms, such as headaches and fatigue, which the researchers did not find. However, their attention levels plummeted, a symptom that persisted for up to a week. Disrupted attention may lead to learning difficulties for kids in school, the investigators warned. The best way to prevent this, they advised sensibly, is to have children avoid highly caffeinated drinks.

Like a bloodhound on the scent, consumer advocate Ralph Nader was on this track over thirty years ago. In a 1969 hearing before a government Committee on Nutrition and Human Needs, Nader issued a dire warning about Coca-Cola. Concerned about the drink's complete lack of nutritional value, combined with its worldwide popularity, Nader argued for a more healthful alternative to calorie- and caffeine-rich Coke, which he called "a massive affliction that someday may be characterized as a disease."

That day has come. Not exactly as Nader prophesied (a global pandemic of "Coca-Cola-ism"), yet close. There is now a medical disorder, "caffeinism," whose symptoms include insomnia, restlessness, and trembling, which is caused by excessive consumption of cola, coffee, and other products. *Caffeinism*: when I first came across the word I thought it sounded absurd—a self-conscious stepchild to *alcoholism*, born of Starbucks. But then I saw an unforgettable report on the TV news regarding "caffeine risks" and consumer efforts to enforce stricter product labeling of caffeine content. To humanize the story, a reporter interviewed an older man who was hospitalized for a simple hernia operation. This patient had two IV drips, one with the standard electrolyte solution, the other with liquid caffeine. His doctor had prescribed it to alleviate symptoms of caffeine withdrawal following the surgery.

"Smoked for twenty-five years and finally quit," the man admitted dolefully, dark circles under his eyes. "But I never had as hard a time as I did trying to stop coffee. Just couldn't kick it."

At bedside, his nurse fingered the IV line and said comfortingly, "Yeah, you've got the equivalent of five cups of joe pumping through you right now." The patient looked with longing at the IV bag, as if he'd prefer to slash it open and drink it. This was, without question, a portrait of advanced caffeinism.

Having traded in my boyhood love of Coca-Cola for an adult addiction to coffee, I could have been looking into my own face twenty years from now—the foreshadowing of a horrible end. Although it's rare, one can even die from caffeine poisoning, scientists say, the acute lethal dose in adults being roughly five to ten grams. Consuming the equivalent of, say, two hundred bottles at once would result in death by Coca-Cola.

⤫

My whole family exhibited signs of caffeinism. Or did we? At this distance, it is hard to say whether it was Coca-Cola or my father who made us so jittery. Perhaps it was a combination of the two, intensified by the ordinary pressures of a big family. By day, we were as orderly and well-mannered as Spokane itself. By night, we were a house of jangled nerves. After Dad came home, chores had to be finished, dinner made, the house picked up. It was always tense in that first half hour, from five-thirty to six. On a typical evening, Dad was stationed in his easy chair, watching the news, drinking a Scotch and soda, while Mom was in the kitchen supervising the girls. Spats erupted among my sisters. Dad demanded silence. As often as not, one of the girls ended up with a swatted bottom.

I can see myself slipping off at such moments for a nice, cool bottle of Coca-Cola. I follow a simple path: from my bedroom, down the hall, through the TV room past Dad, into the kitchen, down the basement stairs, and finally to the refrigerator in the rec room. With bottle in hand, I return to the foot of the steps where, to one side, four shelves display Coke memorabilia. In the basement's dim light, I see empty Coke bottles from around the world (Russia? Mexico?), the familiar white swoosh of the logo beneath foreign letters. Beside them, bottle caps, coasters, and Coca-Cola serving trays are neatly arranged. A golden Coke bottle, a sales trophy of some kind, gleams. I know that it's probably spray-painted, but it looks extraordinarily valuable. Magazine ads from the forties and fifties (". . . the Pause That Refreshes") are in frames on the wall, alongside old black-and-white photos of Mom and Dad.

Though I'd absorb the facts and dates over time, the photographs provided a visual chronology that even a young boy could follow. Clowning for the camera, Mom is sitting in a lifeboat—bare legs and arms akimbo—on the deck of a ship bound for Europe in 1949. She's on her postcollege grand tour. Dad is in dress grays in a portrait taken that same year, at his graduation from West Point. Later shots show him in combat gear; he landed in South Korea in August of 1950 and took part in the first drive north. At first glance, one eight-by-ten seems to be an abstract image taken in a rainstorm. It's actually a cloudy sky full of paratroopers, my father floating somewhere among them. Another shows him saluting as he receives a Bronze Star and a Purple Heart for wounds received in combat. One eye left blind, he's wearing dark glasses.

Next, I see Mom in 1951. She's wearing a full, pleated skirt and cardigan and poses in the apartment she shared with several girlfriends in Manhattan. Shortly after, she's seated next to Dad, in an early photo of the two of them. Introduced by mutual friends in New York City, they're in a nightclub, squeezed between others on a banquette. My father loved jazz, a fact I tend to romanticize: I imagine they're at a downtown club listening to Miles Davis. The table is a mess of pleasures—steak, wine, cigarettes. Dad is as handsome and photogenic as the young and clean Chet Baker. Mom's sleek, dark hair is bobbed. She wears a sleeveless, black cocktail dress; Dad's arm circles her shoulders. Finally, it's November 14, 1953, a formal portrait: he is in his captain's uniform, she is in her wedding gown.

It's ten years later, almost to the day, in one of the last framed items on the basement wall, a clipping from Spokane's morning paper, the *Spokesman Review*. It's a story about the city's new Coke man. I remember it so well, I can almost make out the smudged newsprint. Wanting to see it again, though, I recently found a copy. Under the headline, there's a thumbnail-sized head shot of my dad. He is thirty-nine, the age I am now. I study it closely, but cannot see my face in his. No features match up. Instead, I inherited other traits, I suppose: his stocky build; his heavy sighs; some of his gestures, the way he'd pull out his wallet or put a hand to his temple while listening. In the photo, my father is unsmiling. He looks like a good, decent man, yet not as tired, not as irritable, as he did at home.

Eight years before Dad bought the Coke business, the previous owner modernized the plant by installing a second full bottling line. The addition of $50,000 of new, faster machinery made the local newspaper in July of 1955. It was viewed as both an outrageous sum and a wise investment. The equipment upgrade was necessary to accommodate larger-size bottles, which in itself was a milestone: the first change of any kind in Coca-Cola's bottle design since 1915. Patterned after the traditional six-and-a-half-ounce bottle, two new models were being introduced across the country. Holding twelve and twenty-six ounces respectively, they were called King and Family Size. Spokane would be the first city in the Inland Empire to have them.

Dad's predecessor, H. T. Raymond, was interviewed by the *Spokesman Review* about the new bottles. When the present design was worked out in 1915, he said, the designer was told to "produce a bottle which can be recognized even by feeling it in the dark. It should be shaped [so] that, even if broken, a person could tell at a glance what it was."

It doesn't sound as if he's only talking about a Coke bottle. His comments bring to mind the intuition one develops within a family. With eyes closed, I could recognize my father by the way he cleared his throat or by his jaw popping (another trait he and I share) when he ate Grape-Nuts each morning. It wasn't so much what he said but the look on his face that made an impression. I could gauge his mood the moment he stepped through the door after work. At night, lying in bed listening, I could recognize his faint snoring, then the mattress creaking as Dad got out of bed. His knees cracked as he walked up and down the hallway.

⮞

Presiding over a pop factory was stressful, exhausting work, particularly in a region where the really hot, Coke-drinking weather was limited to two months in the summer. Negotiating with the labor union was enough to keep Dad awake many nights. Expensive trucks broke down; equipment had to be replaced, payroll made, product delivered throughout eleven counties in two states. Of course, none of that was apparent to me as a child. Visiting the Coke plant was a fantastic adventure.

Like a Disneyland attraction, the entire premises seemed to be animated. On the front lawn, an enormous, round clock revolved atop a spindly pedestal. It looked to me like an unblinking eye, calmly watching the traffic on Monroe Street, glancing at the whirring pop factory behind. Visible through windows running the length of the building, bottles raced by on a roller-coaster ride of steel machinery. First, empty bottles were cleaned in a shower of soap suds. They vanished, only to reappear moments later, rinsed, dried, and cooled, filled with a shot of foaming pop. Brown, orange, red, green, or purple, the bottles lined up to be capped, like hundreds of obedient glass soldiers.

In one of the earliest visits I remember clearly, Mom and I dropped by the plant on a weekday afternoon. Inside the front door, a Coke bottle as big as a five-year-old stood sentry. Wow, what lucky kid would get to drink that? I thought. Nearby, people with appointments waited on a shiny wooden bench. With all of the windows, it was warm and sunny. We were greeted by "the girls," as Dad called them, four secretaries seated in the front corner office. "Hello, Mrs. Hayes!" they sang out. "Little Billy!" Two of them would work for Dad for many years to come: a young, bubbly brunette, Nadine, who took care of the books, and an older woman with bleached-blond hair, Rose, who was his assistant. They crushed their cigarettes in ashtrays and got up from their desks to come chat.

No other women worked there. To go into the Coke plant proper was to enter a world of men. The air carried the scent of wet concrete, pop syrup, perspiration, diesel fuel, and tobacco. Walking through that final doorway was crossing over. Machinery and voices were punishingly loud. The cool, windowless corridor, which led to offices on the left, the bottling plant on the right, and a warehouse at the far end, was filled with workers. Men on break hung out there, smoking near a water fountain, punching in or out at the time clock. As we passed through, I remember one guy crouching down to my level and, to my delight, whistling into an empty Coke bottle. Even as a little boy, I could tell what they did—or at least, in which part of the building they worked—by what they were wearing. The salesmen wore suits and ties like Dad. The factory crew wore white coveralls. The drivers wore gray-and-red Coke uniforms.

A man named Lee Talley was the national president of Coca-Cola when my father had purchased his franchise. "Two things make this business great," he said at the time. "One is the product Coca-Cola, and the other is men. We have the product but we shall need more and more good men. Men of character and intelligence. Men who are industrious and hardworking. Men of spirit and ambition. Men of dedication."

Talley's statement sounds like a personal invitation to my father. The Coca-Cola plant must have been a deeply appealing place for him—a big garage of undiluted masculinity.

Teams of uniformed men worked together, united in purpose, while also competing against Spokane's Pepsi-Cola distributor. Reminiscent of being in the army, it combined strategic thinking with manual labor, and Dad was in charge. A child of the Depression and a product of the World War II era, he believed in everything that Coca-Cola itself represented—America, tradition, family, the rewards of hard work, free enterprise.

Dad's office was at the end of the hallway. He had his own Coke cooler, like in our basement, yet it was smaller and offered the promise of surprises. Standing on a chair, I'd stare down into the rows of bottles as if I were contemplating a big box of refrigerated crayons. Sometimes I would spot a drink with a cap and color never seen before—Raspberry Crush, say, or a chocolate-flavored soda—sent to Dad to taste-test and possibly add to the bottling line. I'd take a sip, I'd give him a couple swigs. He'd act as if the decision, yes or no, were mine.

His office also contained a safe. Memory may be playing tricks, but I could swear it was hidden behind a picture on the wall. Like most little kids, I was fascinated by the allure of a closed door (my mother's locked jewelry box was especially tantalizing) and anything having to do with secrets—riddles, magic tricks, stories about buried treasure, games like hide-and-seek. It was a thrill to watch Dad open his office safe.

"Shhhhhhh," he would say with a wink, a finger to his lips, as Mom closed the door. We stood in church silence as he slowly spun the combination—right, left—a dramatic glance over his shoulder (would he remember the final number?)—right—and, finally, unlocked it. He was probably just getting a spare set of keys. His hand shot in and out before I could see past it. But I came to believe, as gravely as I believed in the Devil, that his safe contained a valuable document: the secret formula for Coca-Cola.

There was great mystique surrounding the ingredients, not only as it was playfully encouraged by my father. Part of the drink's grip on American culture had to do with its secret recipe: one that could be approximated but never duplicated; that was guarded like nuclear arms codes; and that few people on the planet were entrusted to know. It was rumored among my sisters and friends that no one really did know, Dad included. Either there was an endless supply, mixed up a hundred years ago in Atlanta, Georgia, or it was capable of a pop form of transubstantiation. As wine was turned into the blood of Christ, so, too, water in a drum became Coca-Cola.

In truth, my father bought premixed Coke syrup directly from the parent company. I figured that out by the time I'd learned to ride a two-wheeler. And the formula wasn't so sacred that they wouldn't later try changing it—a disaster as it turned out—to better compete with Pepsi. But when I was five, things were wonderfully uncomplicated. All I knew was that Dad was the Coca-Cola King and I was his only son. One day, he'd pass on to me the combination to his office safe and the secret of Coke.

Chapter 5

Making a Bed

MOM MEASURED out Dad's morning coffee the night before. A white enamel percolator with a glass eye on top, the pot was always ready when he awoke. He plugged it in and coffee started blinking. The one thing he had to make himself was a bowl of cereal. Dad, who went to mass most mornings, was gone by six. Mom was more of a late sleeper. I might already be up, playing with Matchbox cars, when she came into the kitchen and turned on the light. She'd find me propped against the refrigerator; I liked its warm, ventilated air blown from underneath, its whispery hum. In her housecoat and slippers, Mom made breakfast and bag lunches, then a fresh pot of coffee for herself. She sat down to have her first cup and a cigarette as she wrote a grocery list. Sometimes she ate half a grapefruit, frosted with sugar, or a piece of cantaloupe with salt.

My older sisters ran in and out, needing help with ponytails or braids or zippers on dresses. With a loud knock, the Carnation milkman appeared at the screen door. A tall, fat, laughing man, he looked like an off-season Santa Claus, with a flushed face, glasses, and an easy name like Ned or Fred or Bud. He brought daily bottles of milk, weekly cartons of ice cream—vanilla, Neapolitan, and chocolate-strawberry in a checkerboard design. Mom sent the girls off to school at Comstock. Our baby-sitter took care of four-year-old Julia. After dropping me off at Westminster's for kindergarten, Mom would buy groceries, run errands, then pick me up after lunch.

Once a week she got her hair done. A woman in another neighborhood—a divorcée, I later figured out—had a beauty parlor in her house. The salon was in the basement, down a flight of moss-covered outdoor steps: a small room in which two or three ladies under dryers smoked and talked; chemicals fouled the muggy air; a radio crackled; the hairdresser's laugh and loud voice rose above all the noise. Shabby as an unsewn hem, the parlor's green-and-gold wallpaper peeled at every seam. I watched Mom get a shampoo and set and emerge with a hairsprayed helmet. It did not strike me as a place one would return to willingly.

We were home before my sisters were out of school. Julia and I followed Mom around as she did housecleaning, starting in the basement and working her way up. Now and then, she had hired help—a German woman, Mrs. Hassler, who'd bring a loaf of homemade rye bread as hard as a turtle's shell—but usually Mom was on her own. The washing machine was always running, as if it actually kept our house going, like a big rickety generator. Some days, my mother spent all afternoon downstairs ironing. I can picture the daunting pile of bleached white shirts, handkerchiefs, towels, pillowcases; *Match Game* on TV; Mom's hands moving quickly, pressing out the fabric, taking a drag on her Pall Mall, a sip of Tab, spritzing water from a Coca-Cola bottle. A puff of steam shoots from the iron as she blows out smoke.

I would help her with the dry bedsheets hung on the clothesline outside, holding an end as she unclipped them. "Oh, lands!" she'd say every time. "Smells so good!" And we'd bury our faces in the sweet fabric. As she put up wet sheets, I'd play on the lawn, which was bordered by pine trees that shed all over the yard. I'd braid together dried pine needles, like thick strands of brown hair, or turn piles of them into patterns on the grass. My sisters taught me this craft, something I can now imagine kids doing in Appalachia. With the meticulousness of an autist, I'd design elaborate, multiroom pine-needle houses, as big as the backyard. Each room was "drawn" two-dimensionally—with indications for the door, window, bed—in narrow lines of needles. These were as ephemeral as sand castles—blown away or raked up by Sat, the Asian man who mowed our lawn.

Over an afternoon, I'd wander inside and out as Mom continued cleaning the house, with Julia tagging behind her. In truth, it was never really a mess. When I envision it now, I can't see anything underfoot. It's not that we didn't have stuffed animals, board games, Lincoln Logs, but that we did not leave them out. Dolls were kicked into closets; books shoved under beds; all was hidden from view. We were lucky to have a house that had been designed like a Japanese tansu chest—compartments within compartments, room after room. The main hallway was lined with sixteen drawers of different sizes. In the basement, sliding doors concealed floor-to-ceiling shelves against an entire back wall. Every item had a place, and a name: the game cupboard was in the TV room; the costume box in the basement; crayons were kept in a round tin by the laundry sink; gum had its own kitchen drawer. Even the backyard was remarkably neat. Outdoor toys—balls, rackets, jump rope—were put in a basket in the garage.

A bed was not often left unmade. If so, it looked like a serious mistake: an untidy embarrassment of crumpled bed-spread and wrinkled sheets. My older sisters were expected to make their beds and straighten their own rooms, among other domestic chores, from which I was excused. Setting the din-ner table, clearing it, loading the dishwasher, unloading it, dusting, sweeping, polishing silver, hand-washing china, vacu-uming: these were the province of my sisters and mother. "Squaw's work," as Dad would say. Which made the two of us, I was later to understand, honored guests in our own home. Each week, the girls were assigned a letter, A through D, which corresponded to specific tasks recorded in Mom's date-book. To them, it was proof of indentured servitude. Excluded, I wished only to be part of it.

The final stop on Mom's cleaning rounds was the master bedroom. She'd begin with the bathroom, a cool, rose-colored chamber, like the inside of a conch shell. My baby sister and I stayed out of her way as she scrubbed the tub and pink-tiled floor. Julia toddled off while I poked through Dad's clothes closet in the hall. The floor was a rock garden of black and brown dress shoes. I would clear a space and sit down. The strangely delicious scent of shoe polish—a fragrant mix of dark chocolate and gasoline—drifted from a latched wooden box. I breathed it in and tipped my head back, eyes closed. The pointy ends of Dad's hanging neckties tickled my face— hundreds and hundreds of them, I'd have guessed.

This last memory prompts a whole cluster: my parents are dressing for one of their many evenings out—say, cocktails at the Prosperity Club (a place, I imagined, where the tables were heaped with coins) followed by dinner at the Spokane House. As they're getting ready, the bathroom door's open, kids are welcome; a gathering far more relaxed and intimate than a family meal. I see myself cross-legged on Dad's valet stand in the far corner of the L-shaped room. Mom, in a slip, is seated on her wicker bench in front of a big mirror. She hums to the radio while rummaging through a shallow drawer crowded with lipstick tubes and finally pulls out a small glass bottle. She rubs some beige-colored cream onto her cheeks. Margaret starts testing Mom's different perfumes on Shannon, who's been trying on gloves—Mom has so many pairs, they have their own drawer. Julia's sitting on the floor of Mom's closet petting the mink stole. Colleen, the eldest at age thirteen and our baby-sitter for the evening, stands in the doorway while Mom gives her last-minute instructions: "There's a TV dinner for each of you in the freezer downstairs—three-fifty for forty-five—top oven." Colleen stalks off.

Dad, who'd slipped away for a ten-minute nap in the bedroom, now walks into the bathroom in his boxers and undershirt. He's in a good mood. "Out, out, out, outcha go," he says to Margaret, Shannon, Julia, and me. "Gotta take a shower." He pulls a pair of wing tips from under the valet stand. "Ellen? Where's Ellen?" he says. "Billy, tell Ellen I'll give her four bits if she'll shine these." Ellen's the only girl who's good at shoe-shining. "Diane? Did you give Colleen the number for the Spokane House? Fifteen minutes. Fifteen minutes, Diane, and we've gotta go." He rounds the corner to start the shower as we file out of the bathroom.

"Yes, Pat," Mom says and closes the door.

After Mom finished cleaning the bathroom, I'd watch her tidy up the bedroom. I sat atop the love seat, behind which Shannon and I would sometimes hide when Mom and Dad were out of the house. Shannon and I shared both a bedroom and a special camaraderie at this age. The love seat was covered in plum-colored velvet; its broad back was the perfect surface for a game of tic-tac-toe. We'd trace our X's and O's against the fabric grain. Then, with a wave of the hand, the game was erased. Mom worked the same kind of magic with bed-making. Tossing aside the heavy quilt, she'd wedge their twin beds apart and make them up within seconds. Just as quickly, she'd push the mattresses back together, replace the bedspread, and smooth the wrinkles with her hands, as if it were cake frosting. It looked effortless, but wasn't. A government report from that time estimated that the average American woman walked four miles and spent twenty-five hours per year making and remaking a single bed.

❧

"A truly civilised standard should be one bed, one person, and if possible, one bed, one room. Married people can't expect that, you may retort. Why not? They should do so if they see a good deal of each other and they want to keep the fresh intensity of their love."

Do you recognize this prickly voice? No? Allow me please to introduce Marie Carmichael Stopes, a British doctor of science and philosophy.

It is 1956, the year my mother had her second child, Ellen, and Dr. Stopes is speaking—well, pontificating actually, as is her style—from the pages of her latest book, *Sleep*, just published in the United States. *Sleep* sums up her opinions about all things related to the title subject, from proper pillows to insomnia to sex. She is seventy-five years old, a celebrity in Great Britain and known throughout the world. Trained as a botanist, she wrote one of the first books for women on contraception, *Married Love*, published in 1918, and three years later opened the first birth control clinic in the British Empire. A leader of the birth control movement, she spread her progressive views on "sexology" through a newspaper column,

"Dear Dr. Stopes," in addition to writing twenty-nine scientific books, a play, memoirs, and several volumes of poetry.

With the publication of *Sleep,* Dr. Stopes hopes to shake some sense into the average American housewife. While she'd applaud that my parents have twin beds, for example, she would disapprove of their being smooshed together. "The twin bed set was an invention of the Devil, jealous of married bliss," she proclaims in the chapter "Beds and Bed-Clothes." To keep sexual passion alive, she recommends that each spouse sleep in a separate bedroom, with the wife's room designated as the "romantic place."

Mindful of economic realities, Dr. Stopes understands that "the miserable little shanties . . . being built now" force most couples to share a bedroom. With that said, she turns the page, moving on to a matter of equal gravity. "Consider," she quietly demands, "the making of a bed." Her discourse starts with the bed's equivalent of underpants: "An under-blanket is round the mattress, and this is generally a rather worn blanket, washed many times, so that it has lost its pristine fluff. This is the first foolishness." Which is followed, naturally, by the first Stopes commandment: "Buy a *new* small, fluffy blanket as the under-blanket. You will be surprised how great is the extra comfort it makes."

Next, comes the undersheet. "It is stupid of the house-wife to accept sheets too short and narrow to tuck in properly," she scolds. "Sheets must be large enough so to be tucked as to keep smooth all night, and not to ruck into uncomfortable ridges if the sleeper turns." An extra eighteen inches of length and width is required. When it comes to the flat sheet, silk-worm silk is the doctor's first choice, though linen is an acceptable substitute.

"There are people who advocate flannelette sheets. I think they are detestable." One might think she is referring to flannel advocates themselves, but no: "There is a horrid physical nature in flannelette that gives it a false warmth by lack of ventilation," she continues, "and the stuffiness and perspiration so induced are sheer misery and sleep-destroying."

If wisdom comes with age, so apparently does a militant attention to detail. "After the sheets come the blankets, which also must be sufficiently long and wide," Dr. Stopes notes. "Some people have two, three or even more blankets piled on top of each other because the sleeper 'can never keep warm.' Often this is because they are never properly tucked in." She practically snickers at these ignorant souls. "If only housewives understood this!" she despairs in a kind of stage whisper, then proceeds to explain the correct methodology for tucking.

Last, like a full-length fur coat tossed over the shoulders, comes the "eiderdown" or quilt. Bringing to bear both her training in philosophy and a poet's love for metaphor, Dr. Stopes saves her finest rhetoric for this article of bedclothing. "Does it stay on the bed of even the quietest sleeper? Almost never. One turn of the sleeper is enough to start it slowly, slowly slithering, and it ends up on the floor. The sleeper is awakened by the consequent cooling of his bed. He may lie semi-conscious that he *ought* to retrieve it but has not the will-power to do so, and hence lies without refreshment for hours that should have been spent in deep sleep. Or he gets up and replaces the eiderdown and sleeps again. But his sleep has been broken and a broken sleep has not the same quality of nourishment as deep undisturbed sleep."

Dr. Stopes portrays the battle between a sleeping man and the "slyly wandering eiderdown" as though it were the myth of Sisyphus, retold night after night after night. Ah, but she has a method for gaining the upper hand: sew a width of unlined silk along either side of the quilt and tuck that in with the bedclothes. "Then the sleeper can sleep without disturbance by migrant coverings." In closing, she has one last word for housewives: "It may be difficult to clean under the bed, but it is most important to do so frequently."

Though Marie Stopes comes off now as laughably high-hatted, in her time she was truly a crusader to empower women. Through books such as *Radiant Motherhood*, she encouraged women to take responsibility for their bodies; to make sensible decisions about the number of children they wished—and could afford—to have; and to become experts in their own domain, the home. Even so, her writing sounds like hectoring to me—a voice of authority that's more dogged than "Hints from Heloise" and the messages tucked into all the women's magazines my mother read—*Good Housekeeping, Woman's Day, Ladies' Home Journal*. As if a husband's expectations of a well-run household were not enough!

It seems to me that my mother, trained as an artist and an aspiring painter as a younger woman, was highly skilled on her own. When I was in junior high, she helped start a free art school for children in Spokane; it's still operating today. She was good with her hands, always making things. Not only motherly crafts, such as the birthday-party piñatas she made for every child, and motherly duties, such as extracting splinters, but things for herself. After the kids and Dad were in bed, the kitchen cleaned, laundry folded, and coffee prepped for morning, she often worked at an old black-and-gold Singer sewing machine in the basement.

She'd sew clothes late into the night for my sisters and herself (never, as I recall, for Dad or me). It wasn't really a matter of saving money. She wasn't an insomniac. And I don't believe she was consciously avoiding her bedroom. I think she simply enjoyed the puzzle of building a dress from scratch and the quiet satisfaction that came with it. Left-handed—a characteristic that connoted special, artistic significance but wasn't passed on to any of us—she had her own left-handed scissors and pinking shears. They were never misplaced because no one else could use them. Her sewing table was a mess—a permissible, inviolable mess, I see now—cluttered with spools of candy-colored thread, pin cushions, bags of buttons, an ashtray, peppermints. She worked under a faux-stained-glass Coca-Cola lampshade.

If I couldn't sleep, I'd sometimes find her hunched over the Ping-Pong table in the rec room, where fabric was temporarily laid out. A sewing pattern, like crisp, peeling skin, was pinned to it. By morning, the Ping-Pong table would be cleared, a garment ready for ironing. She could have been a dressmaker in another life, maybe a sculptor or carpenter. Though I took home the trophy, it was Mom who actually carved my Pinewood Derby race car. She could, I suspect, have literally made a bed—frame, box spring, and mattress—if given a pattern to follow.

The secret is the innerspring coils, I am told on good authority. A well-made bed is defined by its springs, which must be strong and flexible. Bared, a spring unit looks like modern sculpture: coil linked to coil in an elegant pattern of steel lace. It strikes me as both an ingenious piece of craftsmanship and surprisingly touching, like seeing a skinny, old man naked. I have an impulse to cover it.

I feel similarly solicitous toward Robert McRoskey, the senior proprietor of the McRoskey Airflex Mattress Company in San Francisco, the last remaining factory in the United States where traditional innerspring mattresses are made to order. I've known of McRoskey's since I moved here fifteen years ago; countless times I've passed its Market Street entrance, where a sample mattress lies near the front door during business hours. A sign invites passersby, "Walk On It!" to test for themselves how sturdy the springs are. Now, I've come inside for the first time to see how the McRoskey family makes mattresses.

As Mr. McRoskey leads me on a private tour, the tall, wiry eighty-two-year-old doesn't seem quite sure of his step. He has a slight hunchback, perhaps from bending over his beds for sixty years, or from going up and down the dark, narrow circular stairs that connect the building's four floors. Interrupting his explanation of spring coils, I ask him the source of a booming sound, like rifle shots finding their target. Mr. McRoskey pauses but doesn't react. "Oh, that's down below," he answers calmly. "Box springs." He's entirely used to the noise. At McRoskey's, founded by his father in 1899, they make their own springs, mill their own cotton, and stuff, sew, and ship their own mattresses, which are not sold in any other stores.

The innerspring coil is a relatively recent innovation, Mr. McRoskey tells me. Prehistoric man is thought to have slept on the ground under animal skins, beneath a cover of trees or with a cave for a roof overhead. Most ancient Egyptians slept on simple floor mats. In *The Odyssey*, Homer described a bed Odysseus made for himself after being shipwrecked by Poseidon and swimming ashore: "Not far from the river he found a copse in a clearing. Here he crept under a pair of bushes . . . with their branches so closely intertwined that when the damp winds blew not a breath could enter, nor the rays of the sun penetrate their shade, nor the rain soak through. Odysseus crawled into his shelter, and at once heaped up the dry leaves into a wide bed—the ground was littered with piles of them. . . . The noble, long-suffering Odysseus was delighted with his bed, and lay down in the middle of it, covering himself with a blanket of leaves. And now Athena filled his eyes with sleep and sealed their lids—sleep to soothe his pain and utter weariness."

Every age has its heroes—and its beds. Four were found

in King Tut's tomb, giving an idea of how Egyptian royalty slept: on carved ebony overlaid in gold, with woven leather strips to support the body, and a narrow headrest for a pillow. One of Tutankhamen's headrests looks torturous, and exquisite: Shu, god of the air, is portrayed raising the sky above the earth; the boy king's head would have fallen upon a creamy cloud of hard, cold ivory. The tomb also contained what might be described as a travel cot for the Pharaonic Age, a precursor to the convertible sofa bed invented in the 1920s. Built of lightweight wood, the bed conveniently folds to one-third its size by means of heavy bronze hinges.

Cleopatra's canopy bed, legend has it, was ornate and comfortably raised off the ground—a suitable site for the queen's extravagant seductions. The reality, however, may have been less than romantic: *canopy* derives from the Greek word for "bed with mosquito curtains." Indeed, in the fifth century B.C., Herodotus described how the fishermen of the Nile slept under their own fishing nets to keep mosquitoes from biting.

A common bed in Saxon times was far from regal—just a sack filled with hay. In wealthy households as well as in poor, sleepers huddled together, privacy forsaken in favor of warmth. An ideal medieval Gothic bed looked like a massive wooden box, impervious to drafts and, one might have hoped, to the Black Death. Trundle beds were a product of the Renaissance: Italian noblemen feared for their lives at night unless a guard was posted at bedside. Rolled out on casters from under the aristocrat's bed, the trundle (or "truckle") bed gave a guard a place to sleep. Louis XIV owned more beds than there are nights in a year; at Versailles, all the frames were made of gold.

A new breed of mongrel furniture appeared in Europe and America in the last half of the nineteenth century: beds that doubled as daytime objects—table, desk, piano, bathtub, bookcase—to conserve space. It was as though sleep itself were dispensable. The Combination Bed and Trunk, patented in 1861, "offered a practical solution to travellers who had difficulty in finding accommodations at short notice," according to its creator. The most famous bed of this era was invented by William Lawrence Murphy in the 1890s: the Murphy bed, which folded up into a closet space, instantly rid a room of its presence.

Around this time, Mr. McRoskey's father got into bedmaking. Born in St. Louis of Polish immigrants in 1879, Edward L. McRoskey moved to California at age nineteen with his older brother. Following a brief apprenticeship in pillowmaking, the McRoskey brothers established their mattress business in the last year of the century. Mattresses at this stage in their evolution were simply coverings made of strong fabric (called ticking) and filled with various materials, from old rags to wood shavings to kapok, a downy plant fiber imported from Asia. For many years, a mattress's bounciness came from animal hair—cattle or hog, but usually from the mane of a horse. Kinked with rubber bands and exposed to steam, "just like women getting a permanent wave," the curled hair functioned "like thousands and thousands of little springs," Mr. McRoskey recalls fondly. "Very nice material, but we can't get a supply anymore."

The bed was revolutionized in the mid-1920s with the invention of the innerspring mattress. Edward McRoskey worked to perfect this innovation, and the design he introduced has not been changed since. A McRoskey spring is crimped, which allows one coil to be snugly hinged to another, forming a helical-lace foundation for the mattress. They are hand-fitted so the springs alternate, clockwise next to counterclockwise, for added stability. As Mr. McRoskey demonstrates, the finished spring unit rolls up as flexibly as a futon. His father named it the Airflex mattress because at the time people were intrigued with the possibilities of air travel. It was right before Lindbergh's flight, Mr. McRoskey remembers; "*Air* was a popular word." Each mattress takes about six hours to make; the company produces an average of fifteen a day; and there is currently a three-month waiting list to get one. "We're working like the devil," he explains, but every detail has to be perfect, down to the ventilator eyelets on the sides.

"It is an art, in a way," he says modestly.

Mr. McRoskey leads me downstairs, where the springs are made. Half a dozen men look up from their work and nod politely. Stepping into the hot, windowless room is like going back in time to the 1940s when the noisy coil-making machinery was brand-new. If it were to break down today, he admits, it could not be replaced. The springs, fashioned from eight-hundred-pound spools of wire, hand-fed into the coiling and crimping devices, are then assembled into various mattress sizes—twin, queen, California king. The spring unit is baked in an oven like an enormous steel sheet cake (this "unstresses" the metal): "Three-quarters of an hour at four hundred fifty degrees," Mr. McRoskey states, revealing one part of what he calls the family's mattress "recipe."

The cement basement walls are covered with writing. What looks to me like crude graffiti turns out to be notes on mattress-making. How much threading wire is required, for instance, to lace an Eastern King mattress, an odd-sized 6'4" by 6'8". I think of these workers' notes to themselves as addenda to the purchase orders the McRoskeys have kept on file for three generations—specifications for every mattress made since 1921. These orders, the heart of the company—making it possible, say, to duplicate the firmness of a customer's thirty-year-old mattress—were just barely saved from a recent fire on the second floor.

At the far end of the basement, the workers are assembling box springs, an invention of the forties. Not having slept regularly on a box spring and mattress since I was a child, I cannot understand why the combination is necessary. Is it just to raise the bed higher? I wonder to myself. Just an added expense? The shots I'd heard upstairs resume, as if now aimed at me. The men are attaching upholstery coils to lumber frames, a loud process that makes it hard to have a conversation, but Mr. McRoskey yells above the din. He says something about how the box spring "responds to your pressure." I hear the words "supple" and "flexible," but even without them I am sold. He speaks about beds with such intensity that his eyes burn. Who am I to question the purpose of a box spring?

The Airflex slogan is "The Mattress That Keeps You Youthful." In fact, the mattress, like the factory and the McRoskey family itself, could not be more oldfangled. The cotton ticking is in the traditional pinstripe, light gray or light blue. "No flowers or wild patterns," Mr. McRoskey says. "Not very glamorous but very practical." On the second floor, a small group of women sew mattress covers with black Singer sewing machines, "bought used in 1921," that look exactly like my mother's. On the top floor, a Garnette machine turns raw Texas cotton into soft, airy "blankets"—the correct term, *batting*, isn't an ethereal enough word for it. The cotton is hand-laid over and under the spring unit, in precise quantities depending upon the firmness ordered, and then the cover panels are put in place. At this point, the mattress is near-to-bursting at its sides and is held together by giant safety pins. Next, it is tied down, sewn up, and finally, tufted, which is like sewing tiny cuff buttons onto an extra-heavy winter coat.

Mr. McRoskey is careful not to make therapeutic claims for his mattresses. Still, he admits, many customers say their bad backs have been cured. As for himself, he sleeps on the softest mattress he sells, an "Extra Gentle." Back on the ground floor, he points out one in the corner. It looks made for a prince, like a sumptuous quilt. I silently pray that he won't ask about my own sleeping arrangements. Would he disapprove of the comfy, old pad of thick foam rubber that serves as my bed or that I share it with a man? Mr. McRoskey is too much of a gentleman to inquire.

Glancing around the showroom, I imagine spending a night alone here—accidentally locked in at day's end by Mr. McRoskey while I'm using the bathroom. Inspired by a book I loved as a child, I've had similar fantasies about sleeping overnight at New York's Metropolitan Museum, in a grand English Renaissance canopy bed. But I'm not so sure that a night at McRoskey's would be equally fabulous. Being surrounded by so many freshly minted beds could be an insomniac hell, each mattress offering a different level of sleepless torment. Would I make it to morning without wise old Mr. McRoskey to serve as my Virgil? Without ever lying down on one of his beds, I say good-bye and leave the mattress factory.

Dr. Kleitman would find all this discussion of beds ridiculous, I am sure. He is of the opinion that beds are a minor consideration in the dynamics of sleep. "The alleged benefits of proper bedspring and mattress have been emphasized," he wrote cynically in 1963, "mainly by the makers of such equipment." Of course, this is a man who confessed he could fall asleep almost anywhere and did. In his experiments, he slept not only in a cold, subterranean cave, but in the discomfort of a U.S. navy submarine and above the arctic circle, where the sun never set (not to mention countless nights hooked up to electrodes in the laboratory). One gets the impression that Nathaniel Kleitman would happily have slept on the ground, covered with leaves, in the bed left warm by Odysseus.

"It is all a matter of likes and dislikes and, except through suggestion, the type of mattress used has little, if any, influence on the 'quality' of sleep." Dr. Kleitman's conclusion has repeatedly been borne out. While many people complain about an uncomfortable mattress, recent studies have failed to demonstrate any difference in sleep quality due to sleep surface. And yet, it's still often easier to blame the bed for the previous night's failings and to buy a new one. It may be the ultimate self-indulgence of the prosperous baby boomer: sleep as a luxury item.

The current generation of luxury beds can be traced to the "Summer of Love," 1968, when Charles Hall, a twenty-four-year-old graduate student at San Francisco State University, funneled plain tap water into a large vinyl pouch. The waterbed was born. Hall's invention became a cultural icon, evocative of youthful rebellion and free love. The gurgling, slurping bed itself sounded as if it were having recreational sex. One model was named The Pleasure Pit. Hugh Hefner reportedly once had a king-size waterbed in the Playboy Mansion covered with the fur of Tasmanian opossum. Loaded with sexual promise, the waterbed also made claims for healthier and more natural sleep, as though in simulation of the womb. But the early, unheated waterbed was rather primitive. Some people said it caused seasickness, flooded bedrooms, and the risk of electrocution. Today's waterbed, on the other hand, is as safe as a Volvo and can be ordered with as many amenities.

Money is no object for some people in search of the perfect night's sleep, and several companies are happy to oblige. The Kingsdown "Passion" collection features the "V.I.P.," a king-size bedset (including both mattress and box spring) that goes for $8,500. It would go beautifully with the "world's most expensive pillow": a 435-thread-count silk case filled with eiderdown hand-plucked from Icelandic duck nests, sold by The Company Store for $2,300. Perhaps the ultimate in pretentious beds is sold by Heals of London, "Outfitters to the Queen": a $10,000 queen-size bedset with a mattress of linen ticking and the curled-horsehair filling that Mr. McRoskey had described. There's something perverse about paying so much for a piece of furniture that is covered up and used in darkness by semiconscious occupants. Nevertheless, I've concluded that insomniacs truly deserve the best, most-luxurious beds, for we are more often awake to appreciate them.

For other consumers, it is not prestige that appeals but what the Swedish manufacturer Duxiana calls "Advanced Technology In Sleeping." In the category of information overload, Serta recently introduced its Perfect Night Sleeper "Vitalize," a $5,000 bed that can be hooked up to a computer; it lets sleepers record their heart rate, respiratory activity, and how many times they move. The bedroom becomes an in-home sleep laboratory. *Who sleeps better? You or your partner?* "When you wake up," a Serta representative tells me, "you get a printed readout of how you slept." Of course, this data would be helpful—even lifesaving—for those with disorders such as obstructive sleep apnea. However, for sleep-troubled people like me, adding test anxiety into the nightly mix probably isn't such a good idea.

One would think that, in this age of technological marvels, a bed that makes itself would be invented—no different from an automatic coffeemaker. You get up, press a button, and sheets snap into place; pillows are fluffed; bedspread smoothed. It may be the kind of thing that only a housewife dreams about. Or a kid. Making a bed seemed like a big job when I started out at age six. Mom taught me how; Dad inspected my work. The first occasion was during the summer between kindergarten and first grade, when my parents moved Shannon in with Julia, converted the twin beds into bunk beds, and the room became mine alone. It marked a transition, in the same way that learning to tie laces changes a child's relationship to his shoes. One morning, my bed became something other than a place to sleep. My bed became a responsibility.

Chapter 6

❧

Good Sleep

T HE METAPHORICAL bed is at least as old as Homer. Near *The Odyssey*'s end, Odysseus prepares for bed—to sleep with his faithful wife, Penelope, for the first time in twenty years—only to find that the bed itself is the test of his true identity. Wary of being deceived by the gods, Penelope forces Odysseus to reveal the "great secret" of their marriage bed, known only by the two of them. Building it "was my work and mine alone," Odysseus says, describing a bedpost carved from the trunk of a living olive tree, around which he had built their bedroom. Immovable, literally rooted to the earth, the bed is the center of their home, symbolic of their love for one another. Penelope bursts into tears and finally kisses him. The secret of the bed, rather than Odysseus in the flesh, has provided the "infallible proof" that he has returned. At that, a housekeeper puts "soft bedclothes" on it and "blissfully they lay down." The Greek critic Aristophanes claimed this scene was Homer's original end to the poem, with the subsequent lines added by a later writer. It seems fitting. What sweeter reward than to sleep in one's own bed after surviving the Trojan War, Cyclops, the wrath of Poseidon? What happier ending?

In life as in myth, truth is told in bed. Relationships are put to the test, but also strengthened. Comfort is psychic, not just physical; spiritual as well as sexual. Can you fully trust the person with whom you are sleeping? How well do you know the body sharing your apartment or dorm room or barracks or house or jail cell? Or are you the dishonest one, like the unnamed "evildoer" in Psalms 36 who "plots mischief while on his bed"? Take heed, as the Old Testament prophet Micah warned: "Woe to those who devise wickedness and work evil upon their beds!" In sleeplessness you may suffer.

For the insomniac, bed is a place of reckoning. In darkness, one's conscience is examined, deeds assessed, shame felt. Unable to sleep, King Ahasuerus in the Old Testament Book of Esther arrives at the decision to honor Mordecai, which saves him from the hanging secretly planned by Haman. King Ahasuerus then hangs the evil Haman instead; the Jewish people are saved through an episode of biblical sleeplessness. Job also suffered insomnia, in addition to his many tragedies: "When I lie down, I say, 'When shall I arise?' But the night is long, and I am full of tossing till the dawn." Beyond hope, Job envisions his fate: "The grave is mine house: I have made my bed in the darkness."

The notion of a "bed of justice" originated in the fourteenth century. It literally denoted the bed upon which the king of France reclined when present in Parliament: *lit de justice*. From this original meaning, the expression came to signify Parliament itself. It might also explain the source of a proverb used throughout the world, in which the state of one's bed reflects the state of one's life: "As you make your bed, so you must lie upon it." Similarly, it is said that peace of mind is an honest person's pillow. On the morning President Clinton was impeached, he cited his seven hours' sleep as the best evidence of his untroubled condition.

You ultimately get what you deserve in bed, one may believe, depending upon how you've led your life or behaved that day. For a child, few punishments are harsher than being sent to bed without supper. In Maurice Sendak's *Where the Wild Things Are*, Max's mischief lands him in this loveless, famished state, from which his wicked fantasy grows. Like Dorothy to Oz, he travels far from home. After he tames the Wild Things and is made king, Max sentences them to the same punishment he'd received from his mother. Lonely, hungry, he then gives up his throne and happily sails back to a hot supper, waiting for him in his own bedroom. There may seem no safer, more comforting place. To be loved and cared for, read to, tucked in, kissed good-night, and wished "Sweet dreams" is to feel that all is right with the world. And that sleep—good sleep—is effortless. But what is "good sleep," for child and adult alike? How does one get it?

The unmistakable stench of a burnt coffeepot is in the air when I consult Dr. Dale M. Edgar in his paper-strewn office. A highly regarded neurological researcher at Stanford University, he could be describing me as he says, "People think of sleep and wakefulness like a light switch. This stems from childhood—when it's 'night-night' time, you flick the switch off, kerplunk, you go to sleep, and you tend to think in similar terms. We talk about 'the moment of sleep,' that instant in which you go from cognitively aware to less cognitively aware.

It's actually a continuum." According to a theory he's developed, "There are neurobiological functions that drive you toward sleep and others that act to oppose it." The two "battle" one another in a portion of the dime-sized hypothalamus, the suprachiasmatic nucleus (SCN), where the brain's master biological clock is located.

"It's not a switch, it's a war," Dr. Edgar states, his boyish face lighting up with enthusiasm. "You can think of these two functions as sabers, fighting it out." I half expect him to pull action figures from the desktop clutter to help him demonstrate. "During the day," he continues, "the biological clock is winning," while at night, "the Darth Vader of darkness has taken over and dominates the brain."

I can't help noticing that he has taken sides, with sleep as the archetype of evil. He shrugs and laughs: wakefulness is his specialty. "Darth Vader is *real*," he informs me, smiling broadly; "it's not a vacuum of the White Knight of wakefulness. The sleeping brain is not turned off. Its functions and behaviors can occur as long as the SCN isn't jousting it back."

After a deep breath, Dr. Edgar brings his imagery back to earth. Light cues travel from the eye to the SCN, he explains, triggering "alerting" signals that counter a natural pressure to sleep. These wakefulness signals gradually decrease by nightfall, when the brain begins to orchestrate a complex of sleep mechanisms. Darkness, silence, warmth, satiation, and comfort are critical elements for triggering sleep-inducing neurons, hatched from the lower brainstem. These, in turn, induce slow-wave brain activity. By studying this activity in a laboratory, scientists can determine sleep depth, duration, and whether a person sleeps "efficiently," fully utilizing every minute spent in bed. And yet, while Dr. Edgar's theory of "opponent processes" is generally accepted by the sleep-science community, a definitive answer to how and *why* sleep ends and wakefulness begins—and the reverse—remains unknown.

Before the biological clock was understood and brain waves could be measured—a century before *Star Wars* could serve as a metaphor—a common approach for studying sleep was to observe the conditions under which good sleep occurred. This was an obsession of the Victorian age, when sleep was viewed as a spectral visitor, bringing with it each night coded messages on the state of one's nerves. In fact, some believed that sleep resided in, and rose from, the "tubes" of the nervous system. Sound mental and physical health depended upon good sleep, and vice versa. Therefore, achieving ideal sleeping conditions—"sleep hygiene"—was a vital concern. Scientists such as Marie de Manacéine and others wrote on the subject at great length and with extraordinary passion. We are left with a body of writing that is equal parts philosophy, phrenology, and phenomenology, nineteenth-century public health policy and good-housekeeping tips.

Robert MacNish, a physician in Glasgow, Scotland, detailed his recommendations in an influential early book, *The Philosophy of Sleep*, first published in America in 1834. The "sleeping chamber" should be large and airy, he wrote, "and, if possible, not placed upon the ground-floor, because such a situation is more apt to be damp and ill ventilated." The bed curtains "should never be drawn closely together, even in the coldest weather." I detect no lilting Scottish brogue in his writing voice. Nor do I picture a kind Scottish doctor. Instead, he has the clipped tones of the Queen Mother and calls to mind a character of the same era, Mr. Bumble, the cruel workhouse keeper in *Oliver Twist*.

"The bed or mattress ought to be rather hard," Dr. Mac-Nish dictated, while sitting, I imagine, on a cold, hard bench in a cold, bleak flat. "Nothing is more injurious to health than soft beds; they effeminate the individual, render his flesh soft and flabby. . . . The pillow as well as the bed, should be pretty hard. With regard to the covering, there can be no doubt that it is more wholesome to lie between sheets than blankets. For the same reason, people should avoid sleeping in flannel nightshirts. Such a degree of warmth as is communicated by those means is only justifiable in infancy and childhood, or when there is actual disease or weakness of constitution. Parents often commit a great error in bringing up their young people under so effeminate a system."

Although it sounds absurd and pedantic to my ears, Dr. MacNish's philosophy made sense in the context of the times. As Bruce Haley pointed out in his book *The Healthy Body and Victorian Culture* (1978), sanitation was poor in Great Britain; the water supply was irregular; the brick houses held a "dungeonlike dampness." For every person who died of old age or violence, eight died of specific diseases such as tuberculosis. Nearly a third of infants never reached their fifth birthday. "In an age of mysterious contagions and chronic complaints, when contagions and complaints were part of the same spectrum of ill-health, physicians increasingly turned to hygiene and to the *res non-naturales*—air, water, food, sleep—as the basis of their therapeutics." If the Victorians could not cure diseases, they thought at least they could do something to prevent them before symptoms appeared.

Into this dank, infected atmosphere, British physician Edward Binns introduced a tonic: *The Anatomy of Sleep; or, The Art of Procuring Sound and Refreshing Slumber at Will*, published in 1842. Reputed to be the world's first book printed with the aid of a typesetting machine, it was illustrated with brightly inked etchings, an effect matched by Dr. Binns's writing style. He sounds at times like a carnival barker, enticing readers into the Tunnel of Slumber in tones as genial as MacNish's are grim. "The following plan has never failed," Binns declared, "so far as we are aware."

After 390 pages devoted to case studies of somnambulism and other phenomena, Dr. Binns finally revealed his sleep cure in a single paragraph. Try as he might to make it complicated, though, the Art of Procuring Sound and Refreshing Slumber at Will amounted to nothing more than a deep-breathing exercise. Rest your head on the pillow, close your mouth, and breathe in through the nostrils, the doctor instructed.

"Having taken a full inspiration, the lungs are then to be left to their own action—that is, the respiration is neither to be accelerated nor retarded." Next, the sleeper-to-be must visualize that "he sees the breath passing from his nostrils in a continuous stream, and the very instant that he brings his mind to conceive this apart from all other ideas, consciousness and memory depart; imagination slumbers; fancy becomes dormant."

"Many ways of thus tiring the brain have been proposed," William Alexander Hammond wrote in his own book *On Wakefulness* (1866). "The more irksome they are, the more likely they are to prove effectual." The most successful method Dr. Hammond discovered came from the English romantic poet Robert Southey. To achieve a good night's sleep, Southey thought of "all soporific things,—the flow of water, the humming of bees, the motion of a boat, the waving of a field of corn, the nodding of a mandarin's head on the chimney-piece . . . Mr. Humdrum's conversations, Mr. Proser's poems, Mrs. Laxative's speeches, Mr. Lengthy's sermons. . . . At length Morpheus reminded me of Dr. Torpedo's Divinity Lectures, where the voice, the manner, the matter, even the very atmosphere and the streamy candlelight were all alike somnific." It always did the trick. "Cowslip wine, poppy syrup, mandragora, hop pillows, spider's web pills, and the whole tribe of narcotics, up to bang and the blackdrop, would have failed," Southey concluded, in what reads like Cole Porter lyrics, "but this was irresistible."

The tranquilizing effects of divinity lectures and priests'

sermons have been experienced by many churchgoers, myself among them. Prayer may also induce sleep, as Nathaniel Kleitman cautiously noted in *Sleep and Wakefulness*. In a chapter devoted to sleep hygiene, he cited a story found in Dr. Binns's book, which was first told by Rabelais in the sixteenth century. It concerned "some monks, who, oppressed with wakefulness, resolutely addressed themselves to prayer, and before they had concluded half a dozen aves, or pater-nosters," Binns had written, "they all fell asleep." By gliding right past this anecdote without further comment, Dr. Kleitman made his skepticism obvious. Prayer clearly was not the first technique he would have recommended. He classified it as a "psychological" ritual, like taking a warm bath—useless on its own. You had to *believe* it would make you fall asleep and sleep well.

My earliest memories of bedtime involve kneeling in prayer each night at my father's behest, not unlike a dog trained to sit and bark. "Say your prayers," he'd tell me, dipping into the doorway. He then hovered in the hall, in the corner of my eye, wearing a bathrobe sewn from a thick, gray army blanket covered with military patches. Hands pressed together, leaning against my bed, I did as I was told, of course. I addressed myself to a crucifix above the headboard: "'. . . If I should die before I wake, I pray the Lord my soul to take. . . .'" This gloomy plea expressed nightly could plant horrifying ideas, it seems to me now, in the developing minds of children. Perhaps it is fear of not surviving the night, mixed with fear of a soul-snatching Lord, that manifests, for some, in fear of the dark.

I really had no idea what I was saying, no concept of the words' meaning, but I sensed *why* I was reciting prayers aloud. The devoutness practiced was more in tribute to Dad than to

God. Under his command, ours was a household of high moral seriousness. The forces of Ireland, Catholicism, and the U.S. military shadowed our every move, from baptism on, in doubt and guilt. Something more than good behavior was expected of the six Hayes children: complete self-effacement. At our best, we could be waved off like a hand disperses smoke. A threat of discipline hung in the air, settling in each night like a black cloud over the dinner table. A white, Formica-topped oval, it was a little too large for the kitchen nook where it stood, and a little too small for the eight bodies sitting around it. Everyone had an assigned seat, mine being to the left of Dad, who sat at the end by the screen door.

Oddly, for such a religious family, we did not say grace at mealtime. Dinner was more of a plebe's exercise; echoes of West Point's mess hall. The table was the setting for a "good manners contest" that ran open-ended for years. There was a weekly winner, picked by Dad, but no clear rules. Which is not to say we disliked it. Among six, the competition was spirited; displaying good manners offered a chance to shine, and to earn a prize: a half-dollar, fished from Dad's silver piggy bank. You had to be careful to sit up straight; keep your napkin in your lap; mind your elbows; eat your peas; say "Excuse me." In such a highly charged atmosphere, slipups were calamitous. Accidentally spilled milk brought gasps from us kids, as if radioactive poison had been tipped. It was far worse if the glass fell to the linoleum and shattered. Tears of remorse would begin even before Dad's reprimand.

It is no wonder that my sisters and I found solace in the Holy Sacrament of Penance. After reaching the Age of Reason, at seven, we could each finally go to confession and have a hearing for our impurities. It was more than a Catholic rite of passage, it was a tremendous relief. We were recipients of a decidedly mixed message: to sin was evil, yet to confess was very, very good, the latter being dependent upon the former. It was the kind of arrangement that encouraged a child to tell lies for the sole purpose of being absolved of them, and to make secrets of the truth.

I now recall only traces of the yearlong training that led up to my first Holy Confession in first grade. Since Comstock was a public school, I attended weekly catechism classes at St. Augustine's, which, in hindsight, was quite appropriate symbolically. The parish was named after the author of *The Confessions* (circa A.D. 400), literature's first spiritual memoir. Augustine candidly examined his own past, including his sexual sins, which would later become my forte. A philosopher, he wrote over ninety books in which he challenged established Christian doctrine and reflected on larger questions of faith and existence. I'd like to think St. Augustine had a greater subliminal influence on me than the catechism itself, which I instinctively disliked. Catechism wasn't designed for discussion. It was a question-and-answer format that emphasized yes and no, right and wrong.

The name and face of my teacher is blanked out—the old Franciscan nun did her duty, I imagine, then must have been whisked off to a missionary post in China (it was always China), the Vatican's version of a Witness Protection Program. I can still conjure up fragments of confusing classroom lessons on the three types of sin—Original, Venial, and Mortal, each with its own list of examples—and on the afterlives in Hell or Purgatory where they could lead you. Maybe it's just my self-doubt I recall. I was already well versed in sin's possibilities, at least to the extent of a first-grader's worldview.

We also studied the saints, most of whom I already knew from children's books and Sunday sermons: Augustine, Teresa, Bernadette, Jude, Francis of Assisi, Clare, Aloysius, the girls and boy at Fatima. They seemed more a part of my family than the relatives we never saw, who lived in Minnesota. My father talked about the saints and their stories. One of my sisters had a collection of female saint dolls—each dressed in a gray or black nun's habit, accessorized with a rosary—as though Barbie had dumped Ken and entered a cloistered monastery. Saints led severely perfect lives, often as lonely social outcasts, and died in terrible suffering: these were our role models. There was a patron saint for every affliction, no matter how mundane. You had only to consult *The Lives of the Saints,* like the yellow pages, to find one who might intercede and fix your dilemma.

Surprisingly, there isn't a patron saint of sleep in the Catholic Church. St. Francis went through an early stage of extreme abstinence, depriving himself of sleep and food in part to attain a state of rapturous, if not delirious, communion with God. Teresa did this, too. But, like her, Francis amended his ways. He found exhaustion a poor condition in which to help others—the truly ill, tired, and hungry—and eventually preached an ideal of fitness: rest was to be taken in moderation and with humility. He would have been a good sleep saint, but I think he became the patron of birds.

I have found someone else to nominate. In *The Anatomy of Sleep,* Dr. Binns described several women with a mysterious sleep disorder he called catalepsy. This malady occurred during the day, lasted many hours, and was characterized by complete muscular rigidity, inhibiting speech and movement. Today, catalepsy is recognized as a seizure associated with certain brain disorders. Some 150 years ago, however, Dr. Binns saw it as a divine affliction, in which the body slept while the soul itself became visible. With hushed reverence, the doctor profiled Maria Morl, known as "the Estatica of Caldaro," a young woman whom I, too, could worship. In her, sleep was a miracle.

Estatica's first episode took place in 1832, at age twenty, immediately after she had said confession and received Holy Communion. From then on, it struck every time she took Communion. For up to eight hours she would remain in "seraphic ecstasy," Dr. Binns reported. A witness described her as "kneeling upon her bed, with her eyes uplifted and her hands joined in the attitude of prayer, as motionless as a statue. . . . When in this state, she neither sees nor hears; . . . she is entranced—but it is neither the trance of death, nor the suspension of life, but a sort of supernatural existence—dead, indeed, to this world, but most feelingly alive to the other." On February 2, 1834, according to Dr. Binns's account, stigmata first appeared on her hands and feet and over her heart. For the rest of her life, pilgrims flocked to see the Estatica of Caldaro, enshrined in her bedroom.

A profound Catholic faith was the common denominator in severe cataleptics, Dr. Binns postulated. Domenica Barbagli, age twenty-nine, another of the exotic female specimens he profiled, was said to be "a poor, simple, illiterate girl, with no other instruction than her catechism." Dr. Binns noted that an esteemed acquaintance, the Earl of Shrewsbury, had actually visited her. While acknowledging that she did fall down a flight of stairs at age thirteen, which left her "crippled" and bedridden, Lord Shrewsbury viewed the accident as God's way of bringing Domenica "to her present state of high spiritual perfection." He found her to be extremely pale and emaciated: "Were her eyes shut, she would be a perfect corpse," Lord Shrewsbury marveled. It seems safe to assume that Domenica—"totally unconscious of everything around her"—tranquil though she may have looked, was not asleep but, for all practical purposes, brain-dead.

It is an important distinction. As already noted, a person's ability to awaken him- or herself characterizes sleep, whether it is "sound sleep" that goes uninterrupted or "poor sleep," marked by repeated awakenings. Under the rubric of "good sleep," one finds various types and interpretations through history. For a working definition of "beauty sleep," for instance, I am indebted to Edwin F. Bowers, M.D., writing in the *New York Medical Journal* in 1918. Beauty sleep is "achieved during the hours preceding midnight," he explained matter-of-factly, because it adds to the hours "which, under ordinary conditions, we . . . spend in bed."

Women need half an hour to an hour more "deep sleep" per night than men, who require nine hours, "undiluted by disturbance," Dr. Bowers prescribed. He was equally precise in his rules governing the sleep of children. Younger ones need more sleep than older children. The "vigorous" need less sleep than the "delicate." And all children should get more sleep in winter than in summer. From age six to nineteen, a minimum ten hours of sleep a night is necessary.

H. M. Johnson, Ph.D., a research director at the University of Pittsburgh, took up the subject of good versus bad sleep in *Harper's* magazine in 1928—that is to say, sleep's inherit goodness or immorality. His bias was noticeable with his opening words. "When a person falls asleep he loses most of his personal dignity," he wrote. "He begins to behave much like a vegetable, and he looks the part. Apparently he does nothing, knows nothing, and enjoys nothing until he recovers from that condition."

Dr. Johnson noted that, in his role as a researcher, he received letters from people "whose main interest in sleep lies in the problem of getting along with less of it." Disregarding "communications from cranks and psychopaths," the questions he was most commonly asked were none too different from those people worry about today: How long ought one to sleep? Do people generally tend to sleep too much? To these, one could add the question with which he titled his *Harper's* article: "Is Sleep a Vicious Habit?" In the doctor's professional opinion, yes, it most certainly was.

⮂

Sleep as a vice and wakefulness as a virtue were built into Catholic doctrine. Vigil, a church service held late at night on the eve of a Holy Day of Obligation such as Easter, is an institutionalized form of wakefulness, symbolic of sacrifice and devotion. In the theatrical language of Catholicism, it recalls the Agony at Gethsemane, the night before Christ is crucified. Knowing that betrayal is imminent, Jesus goes to the garden with his disciples. "Sit here, while I go yonder and pray," he says in the Gospel according to Matthew. Upon his return, he finds his disciples asleep. He says to Peter: "So, could you not watch with me one hour? Watch and pray that you may not enter into temptation; the spirit indeed is willing, but the flesh is weak."

Twice more, Jesus returns from prayer and finds his disciples sleeping. Such an instance of sloth, of spiritual indifference, is one of the seven capital sins in Catholicism. The third time, Jesus finally implores: "Are you still sleeping and taking your rest? Behold, the hour is at hand, and the Son of man is betrayed into the hands of sinners. Rise, let us be going." At this, Judas appears. If the disciples hadn't fallen asleep, the gospel implies, they might have saved Jesus.

To reunite with Him in the sacrament of Holy Communion, you had to be free of sin. Therefore, learning how to confess properly was our most important lesson in catechism class. Like toilet training, it took weeks of practice before you could do it alone behind a closed door. We rehearsed the examination of conscience. We memorized new prayers, such as the Act of Contrition, and were coached to speak in a barely audible whisper, a decibel level theretofore unknown to seven-year-olds. You had to speak loudly enough so your sins could be heard by the father confessor, but not by the line of waiting penitents.

A skill mastered in the classroom seldom survived the first time the confessional screen slid back—*fwhoooosh!*—and a dim light streamed in, leaving the sinner exposed in all his guilt and terror. What I remember is momentarily forgetting everything I had learned. The musty air turned rancid with Father Austen's breath, redolent of cigars and alcohol. It was like coming face-to-face with the Devil. Not the Devil shown in the children's missal—a hideous, green-bodied ghoul—but the shape-shifting kind who could assume human identities and walk the earth. With his crew cut, deep monotone, and unsmiling poker face, Father Austen was a living, breathing version of another gruff inquisitor, Sergeant Joe Friday.

"Uh, bless me, Father, um, for I have sinned." In spite of nervousness, those words carried an undeniable thrill. They were the incantation leading to "a clear conscience," a place of the mind so ephemeral it lasted no longer than a nosebleed, yet so intoxicating you endured the humiliation and returned for more. Grace was a temporary pleasure, unavailable at home. Every other Saturday afternoon for many years, Dad drove us to St. Augustine's to get some. Mom—"a designated saint," as Dad proclaimed—never had to go.

He was doing his Catholic duty, as instructed by the Church, introducing us to the "mysteries of the faith." Even so, I cannot imagine regarding children as sinners. Badly behaved, spoiled, willful, mean, troubled, rotten: yes. But riding in the backseat of the station wagon on the way to confession—in silence, as we thought about our misdeeds; Dad's face in the rearview mirror—was to be steeped in shame. It is memorized for life, like the way to church. We had learned that we could not forgive ourselves. Forgiveness could only be granted.

" 'O my God, I am heartily sorry for having offended thee and I detest all my sins because of thy just punishments but most of all because they offend thee.' " My sisters and I would say our prayers of penance, then wait in a pew at the back. Dad would circle the church saying his rosary as he followed the stations of the cross, a reenactment of Christ's path to crucifixion. His devotion was genuine, and mystifying. I can still see him, floating in and out of my peripheral vision: head bowed, on his knees.

⌒

Within a lengthy bibliography of declassified CIA documents, obtained through a standard Freedom of Information request (keywords *sleep* and *dream*), I recently noticed a reference to a memo, dated eight months before my parents were married, the subject of which was a man with the same full name as my father's. The good people at the CIA kindly complied with my urgent request to see it. As the first page of the fax slowly came through, with his name on top, I was struck by a terrified excitement: it described an accused American spy who had undergone a prolonged period of torture in "Red China" in the early 1950s, including extreme sleep deprivation. Released from prison, hoping to go next to North Korea, he recounted his experience in a CIA debriefing. I couldn't tell who wrote this lengthy memorandum—the author's name was blacked out.

"Regarding his success in surviving this agonizing period," the document opened: "He attributes this first to faith." While his Communist captors had used wakefulness as a weapon—depriving him of sleep, as well as food or water, in their "brainwashing" sessions—"Hayes said he had recourse to prayer, and it literally gave him stamina for survival."

I was stunned. The parallels with my father were so eerie as to make me think I'd accidentally stumbled upon the hidden truth about him. My God, I thought, this explains it all: his sleep problems, his moodiness, his penchant for secrecy— all passed on to me. Perhaps it answered other questions, too. Exactly why did Dad make parachute drops into North Korea?

How did he get wounded? And finally, what was the source of his evangelical Catholic faith?

As the fax continued, the story went into further detail. "SECRET," stamped at the top and bottom of every page, had been crossed out. Hayes was able to withstand interrogation, it said, by being "sincere in all that he told the Reds. He said he never lied. . . . He admitted, though, 'There were times I apparently said things that I couldn't remember afterwards having said, and which were false.' He had told untruths, but under a duress that had in it the most sinister aspect of brain-washing."

"Hallucination," Hayes declared, "is part of the Red-imposed confession technique. You're a bit hungry all the time. . . . You're sleepy all the time. You forget things, get them confused. You admit and believe things that never happened, while in this fog." And he noted, "when a person is hungry and sleepy, the implied decrease or increase of rations or sleeping time constitutes threats of the most effective kind."

What was most important, Hayes reported, was "to keep your mind busy so as to survive without actually being brain-washed." This sounded to me very much like a prescription for chronic insomnia. " 'I found certainty in prayer,' Hayes also said."

"I have talked to quite a number of these brainwashed gentry," the memo writer added. "I am convinced . . . that everyone who goes through brainwashing carries traces of it for prolonged periods, or always. This is not necessarily bad; this can be good. What is important is to keep it in mind."

On the sixth of seven pages, my working theory imploded: the two Hayes men were the same in name alone, the other identifiers being either clearly wrong or coincidental. The accused American spy was sixty-five years old in 1953, it said, "a tall, strong-looking man, broad, wearing a beard." He was a Christian missionary, wrongfully imprisoned. His wife was Scottish; they had five children, four born in China. I'll admit, I was disappointed. I had not found my father's darkest secret, but his do-gooder doppelgänger. Neither had I stumbled upon a covert method for surviving insomnia. It was only a vignette from the Cold War, a tale of another man's nightmare in the global battle between democracy and Communism. I had yet to figure out the deeper truths about sleep and wakefulness.

PART TWO

SLEEP AND ITS
DERANGEMENTS

The startling fact was this:
my body was offering a precise physiological equivalent
to what had been going on in my mind.

—Joan Didion
The White Album, 1979

Chapter 7

⤛

Sleepwalking

I RESOLVE TO make another attempt to meet Nathaniel
Kleitman. I know that I have just one slim chance: his
firstborn daughter, Hortense.

With no idea whether or where she lives today, I run the
name Hortense Kleitman through various search engines on
the Internet. Nothing. Her sister, Esther, isn't any help; in a
letter to me, she neither confirms nor denies the existence of
Hortense. The last time she was heard from publicly, so far as
I can determine, was forty-six years ago at age twenty-four. Dr.
Kleitman took his family to the Arctic for a summer to study
sleep in a land without nightfall (a polar version of his Mammoth Cave experiment); he and Hortense then cowrote an ar-

ticle about it for a 1953 issue of *Scientific Monthly.* "She has served her father as a 'guinea pig' since infancy," the magazine noted; "this marks her debut as his coworker."

Maybe she didn't measure up. Maybe she stayed at the North Pole. I entertain the possibility of hiring a private eye but, after making one phone call, conclude it's both too deranged and too expensive. I give her up for dead, tragically killed before her father (cancer, I decide), and then unexpectedly come upon her full married name on a document in the University of Chicago's archives. It even contains Hortense's address—a small town in the Midwest. My fawning, overanxious request to meet her and, perchance, her father—express mailed the next day—elicits a brisk reply: *No.* I could swear Esther forged her signature.

My only consolation: word from a colleague that a videotape exists—an interview with Dr. Kleitman conducted ten years ago, when he was ninety-four. I track down a single copy of the tape at the physiology department at UCLA and make a deal with a secretary to borrow it for a few days, in exchange for $25 plus postage. When the tape finally arrives, I find it's in some unheard-of foreign video format—it was made in Amsterdam or someplace—and has to be converted to VHS. Twenty dollars later, and several years after first encountering Nathaniel Kleitman's work, I put the tape in my VCR and open a Heineken.

There he is, in my darkened living room, sitting opposite me in a wing chair. As the video begins, Esther darts in and out of the frame, patting his shoulder, whispering in his ear, fixing his microphone. I realize, chastened, that if she and her sister didn't wish to assist me, they're just protecting their dad. Looking far less majestic than I'd envisioned—more like a frail resident of the Jewish Home for the Aged—he haltingly answers the off-camera interviewer's questions about his career.

I can barely hear him, the sound is so poor, but it doesn't matter much. In truth, it's not all that illuminating. Then, commenting on the task of writing and updating the two editions of his masterwork, *Sleep and Wakefulness,* Dr. Kleitman does something that takes me by surprise: he expresses heartfelt thanks to his wife and daughters for helping him.

I turn up the volume as far as possible and move closer to the screen. "My family was very devoted to me, whether I deserved it or not," Dr. Kleitman continues. His thin voice has sweetened with affection and humility. At last, I feel I'm getting to see the human side of the legendary father of sleep science. I look the old man in the eye.

"What's a family for?" he muses. "Usually it's for trouble," he says, pausing. "But sometimes it's also for good deeds."

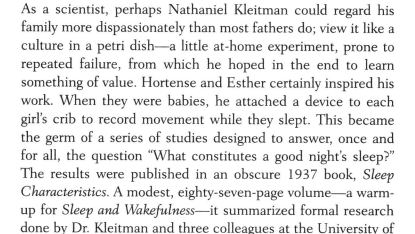

As a scientist, perhaps Nathaniel Kleitman could regard his family more dispassionately than most fathers do; view it like a culture in a petri dish—a little at-home experiment, prone to repeated failure, from which he hoped in the end to learn something of value. Hortense and Esther certainly inspired his work. When they were babies, he attached a device to each girl's crib to record movement while they slept. This became the germ of a series of studies designed to answer, once and for all, the question "What constitutes a good night's sleep?" The results were published in an obscure 1937 book, *Sleep Characteristics.* A modest, eighty-seven-page volume—a warm-up for *Sleep and Wakefulness*—it summarized formal research done by Dr. Kleitman and three colleagues at the University of Chicago.

Theirs was an unusually ambitious study—larger, with more complex variables, and lasting longer than had been attempted before. They examined six sleep characteristics in thirty-six men and women, ages nineteen to fifty-five, with an average of 179 nights' sleep per person. Three characteristics were considered subjective: ease of going to sleep, incidence of dreaming, and the feeling on awakening. Two were objective: motility during sleep and duration of sleep. And one contained elements of both: sleeping continuously. By thoroughly analyzing each of these, Dr. Kleitman and his team hoped to nail down the essential criteria for getting adequate sleep.

As he stated right up front, with charming sincerity, the study was generously supported by a grant from the maker of Ovaltine, which the researchers tested for its sleep-inducing effect against warm milk and tranquilizers such as Amytal and Evipal. There was no conflict of interest, Dr. Kleitman emphasized. In fact, the sleeping tablets were judged the more powerful soporific. Ovaltine, however, did seem to decrease sleep movement, they concluded, whether served hot or cold, in milk or water.

I'll bet the owners of Ovaltine were pleased. At the time, motionless sleep was hailed as the highest-quality rest, something to aspire toward, for it suggested mental and moral soundness. "The longer a person lies still," Dr. H. M. Johnson had written earlier, in 1928, "the more evident it is that he is asleep to . . . [and unbothered by] disturbances, operating upon, and inside, his skin." Of course, some movement was unavoidable, even in healthy sleepers. These alternating periods of quiet and motility follow a curious natural law, Dr. Johnson surmised. Here, I believe, he was closer to the truth: every body has a characteristic rhythm that is peculiar to itself and not easily broken. Sharing a bed with another makes little difference. In sleep, we each move in step with our own internalized restlessness.

Dr. Johnson also sought to determine the ideal position for sleeping. Is it best to sleep on one's back, side, or stomach,

or to employ a broad repertoire of postures? He and two colleagues directly observed 112 sleepers over periods ranging
from several weeks to two years. "It looks as if the most restful
night's sleep is characterized by the use of a considerable variety of bodily positions, all of which are contorted; none of
which indicate anything like 'complete relaxation,'" Dr. Johnson concluded in a 1930 paper for the *Journal of the American
Medical Association*. I think he was disappointed. "To get a
healthy person to spend the night in any one position," he
added, "one would need to strap him to a frame, or else put
him into a cast."

Other scientists would later interpret the behavioral
meaning of various positions. "When we see a person sleeping
upon the back, stretched out like a soldier at attention, it is a
sign that he wishes to appear as great as possible," a British
doctor reported in the medical journal *The Lancet* at the beginning of World War II. He apparently thought he'd found a
clandestine method for weeding out bad men: "One who lies
curled up like a hedgehog with the sheet drawn over his head
is not likely to be a striving or courageous character but is
probably cowardly. A person who sleeps on his stomach betrays stubbornness and negativity."

More recently, a New York psychoanalyst took this a step
further; Samuel Dunkell advised using sleep positions as a diagnostic tool. "In sleep we act out the dramas of our lives,
using our bodies instead of our speech to express our joys and
griefs, our loves and hates," he wrote in his 1977 book, *Sleep
Positions*. "In the night world, each of us becomes the pan-
tomimist of his own personal saga." In what occasionally
sounds more like a guide for drag queen voguing, Dr. Dunkell
identified, illustrated, and named dozens of "exotic" positions,
from the "Ostrich" to the "Clam" to the "Flamingo," each with
corresponding psychological traits. He dubbed the "Barry-
more" after an eleven-year-old boy who was deeply interested

in the theater, a sleep position that could presumably be used to "out" other young Broadway-musical-loving sissies. The boy slept on his side, with "cheek in hand, his arm supporting his head, while the other arm was placed akimbo on his hip." He maintained "this gratifyingly flamboyant position" for a few hours, the doctor noted, before returning to a "normal" position.

In their study of sleep characteristics, Dr. Kleitman's team was interested only in the physiological rather than the psychological significance of sleep positions and motility. To measure movement, Dr. Kleitman invented an apparatus to attach to a sleeping subject's bed, an elaboration of the device he first used with his infant daughters. Studying his hand-drawn diagram in *Sleep Characteristics,* I am struck by the ingenuity of the design: he turned the entire bed into a crude yet effective motion sensor.

A vertical rod transmitted a bedspring's subtlest movements to a large rubber drum, fitted with two valves and placed on the floor. As the drum responded to the compressed bedspring, one valve switched on an electric circuit that caused a clock to start. When movement ceased, the other valve shut off the electricity, stopping the clock. To ensure accuracy, a second electric clock was rigged to stop whenever movement started. By comparing the clocks, Dr. Kleitman could tell how much time the sleeper spent moving during the night, down to the second.

Frequency of movement was counted separately on a saw-toothed wheel clamped to the bed frame. It looked like an accoutrement from a torture chamber. Each time the sleeper moved, the wheel advanced one notch by means of a lever that was connected to the bedspring by a cord, laced through fixed pulleys and counterbalanced by a weight. While the wheel's cranking may have been bothersome to the test subject, like a rattling window, and the electricity coursing under the bed could have been hazardous, the method for recording body temperature was even worse. To test the theory that movement was linked to temperature, subjects slept with a rectal thermometer. Provided with a flange to prevent it from slipping out, the thermometer was connected to a recording machine with a long cord.

Exactly how one slept under these conditions is beyond me. In any event, Dr. Kleitman and his colleagues obtained results. Although they found a decrease in movement after drinking Ovaltine, it did not correlate to subjective reports of having slept well. Body temperature also had no bearing. Nor did the five other study characteristics consistently influence or predict good, quiet sleep. Instead, they varied from subject to subject and in the same individual from night to night. Even under strict laboratory conditions, "good sleep" was irreducible—as difficult to create on command as a perfect child, as reluctant to follow rules as a bad one.

Soon after, Dr. Kleitman packed up his thermometers and rigging and moved on to other areas of sleep research. It's a shame. He might have been on the eve of solving a minor human mystery. What pushes some of us *beyond* the boundary of our beds? When is sleep movement transformed into somnambulism?

All five of my sisters remember me as the family sleepwalker. Shannon recalls helping Mom fold clothes in the den late one night when I appeared. Perhaps it was the fragrant smell of laundry, like incense, that drew me. I stopped in front of the TV in my pj's, eyes open, and began yelling. It was gibberish, Shannon remembers, but the choking anger behind it was alarming. While that behavior alone is odd, the aspect of her story I find most fascinating is my mother's reaction: unfazed. "He's only sleepwalking," she murmured, as though it were as common as the evening paperboy's late delivery. I imagine her then saying calmly, "Okay, Shannon, let's start on the towels."

Mom confirms this scenario. Beginning when I was eight years old, I often materialized before her, an hour or two after I'd gone to sleep. Many times, she says, I walked into the kitchen and quietly stared out the window. In *The Philosophy of Sleep* (1834), Dr. MacNish tells the story of a sleepwalking boy whom witnesses saw leave his home and climb a steep outcrop of rock to where an eagle had built its nest. When he woke the next morning, the boy recalled the incident as only a dream. But, lo and behold, there was the eagle's nest, tucked under his bed. I'd like to think that I was just as daring a somnambulist. Armed with the courage "to walk on the house-top, to scale precipices, and descend to the bottom of frightful ravines," to use Dr. MacNish's words, I picture myself opening the kitchen window one night while Mom isn't looking. I climb out and sleepwalk across Spokane.

My trip is in the fictional tradition of Neddy Merrill, the protagonist of my favorite John Cheever story, "The Swimmer." Nursing gin at a midsummer pool party, Neddy impulsively decides to "swim home" by way of the backyard pools strung across the county. "The only maps and charts he had to go by were remembered or imaginary," Cheever wrote, "but these were clear enough." Neddy says good-bye to his wife, dives into the party host's pool, swims across it, hoists himself out, walks to the neighboring pool, and so on, until he reaches Bullet Park, eight miles to the south. My sleepwalking medium would not be suburban pools, but backyard fences. Nor would I be heading home, but leaving it.

Once outdoors, I get my bearings atop our side gate and scamper to the end of our property. My balance is flawless; I am Olympic material. With new houses being built in the woods behind Comstock Court, every family on the block has also fenced in their yard. I have a straight path across the tall, sturdy pinewood fences bordering the other homes on our street. Like Neddy Merrill on his journey home, I catch back-door glimpses of dramas that normally go unseen. There's the banker's wife, a mother of five who seldom leaves her ornate purple house and wears a black silk bathrobe most days (kids call her "the witch"): bottle in her lap, she's passed out in front of the TV. At the next home: the new neighbor, whose base-ment office walls are papered with *Playboy* centerfolds, is in his young daughter's room; through the window, I can see his shirt is off and she's crying. Farther down, the block's juvenile delinquent is smoking a joint on the patio: for a moment, he thinks he sees me. *"What the hell?"* That's when I hop off, leaving small footprints in the grass like muddy cat paws on a car top. I cross the street, climb onto the next fence and head north, sleepwalking until I disappear.

"No," my mother told me in a recent talk, "I'm afraid you never even made it into the garage." When I press her for de-tails about my sleepwalking—which ended as suddenly as it started, after two years—she is maddeningly short on colorful anecdotes, as is my father. I never walked someplace danger-ous or did anything strange that either can recall. Maybe they're being discreet; sleepwalkers are known to urinate or defecate in inappropriate places. If I did, all is forgiven. As for myself, I remember no more than the vague, morning-after comments from my parents and sisters. I never woke up any-where but in my own room. I never injured myself. I never found anything remotely avian under my bed.

My parents understood that sleepwalking wasn't cause for concern, as long as I made it back to bed without harming myself, which is exactly what a doctor of sleep medicine today would say about it. In general, sleepwalking is considered nor-mal in children. It's more common in young boys and tends to pass by adolescence. About 40 percent of children sleepwalk at least one time; 3 percent do it more than once a month; and 1 percent sleepwalk into adulthood (at which point it is considered abnormal behavior). In the lexicon of sleep, sleepwalking (or somnambulism) is classified as a "parasomnia." Parasomnias are physical phenomena that occur during sleep, including bedwetting, headbanging, teeth-grinding, sleeptalking, and night terrors. Sleepwalking falls into a finer category, "disorders of arousal," which means there is a partial arousal from sleep. In a sense, the person is "caught" between a deep sleep state and full wakefulness.

In its classic form, a sleepwalker's behavior is as stylized and refined (and perhaps as confounding) as minimalist choreography: a Merce Cunningham solo set to a near-silent John Cage score. A very young sleepwalker may simply be heading toward a light source. An older child may have a more independent agenda. He or she may get out of bed and do the same mundane thing repeatedly—fumble with favorite toys, open a closet, get dressed and undressed. It may be a recurring ritual: night after night, a child appears at the foot of her parents' bed or, as I did, goes to the same part of the house.

An episode may last less than a minute or continue for thirty to forty minutes, but will most likely occur in the first third of a night's sleep. Rather than the stereotypic zombie posture—arms uplifted and perpendicular to the body—a sleepwalker appears as if awake, only somewhat clumsy and aimless. The eyes are often open but have a vacant look.

Mystified by the sleepwalker's apparent ability to "see" and walk in the dark, William Alexander Hammond, an American Civil War–era physician, believed the secret was in the sense of touch. Writing in 1869, he observed, "Far from being diminished in its action . . . [touch] is invariably unduly exalted." Dr. Hammond elaborated: "Though the eyes do not see, the ears hear, the tongue taste, or the nose smell, the somnambulist has [this] one sense which is fully awake, and by which he is enabled to guide himself through the most devious passages in dangerous paths." A modern physician would disagree with Dr. Hammond. The fact is, sleepwalkers are guided by memory. They follow familiar paths—to the bathroom, down stairs, into the backyard—that they could negotiate while awake, even with their eyes closed.

A sleepwalker's behavior can be described on a continuum from calm to agitated. If restraint is attempted, an upset sleepwalker may struggle to escape, with unprecedented strength, as though fending off an attack. Vocalizations, if made, are usually unintelligible. Sometimes sleepwalking overlaps with another disorder of arousal: night terrors. Uncommon in very young children, more frequently seen in adults, a night terror may begin with the sleeper bolting upright in bed and screaming bloody murder. The person's eyes are usually wide open; the face is a mask of intense fear. In a full-blown episode, the sleeper may jump out of bed and run blindly, as if from an unseen threat, flailing about, knocking into walls and furniture. As in sleepwalking, none of this activity is remembered upon awakening, typically, any more than one recalls kicking off a bedspread while asleep. Unlike insomniacs, who pay lavish attention to each passing hour—committing it to memory with a mix of grief and nostalgia—parasomniacs are oblivious to time and to their own conduct.

This makes proper diagnosis challenging and statistics somewhat dubious. The prevalence of sleepwalking and night terrors, therefore, may be much higher than has been suggested. In people who report (or rather, who are reported by others to have) chronic episodes, doctors first try to rule out any underlying medical problems as the cause. Sleepwalking may be associated with epileptic disorders, for instance, or a symptom of Tourette's syndrome, but such cases are rare. It's also been linked to breathing disorders, such as obstructive sleep apnea, as well as to migraines. Twenty-eight percent of children who suffer these headaches sleepwalk, one study found.

In Betty Ford's drinking days, Secret Service agents reportedly saw her sleepwalking through the White House. The relationship between substance abuse and parasomnias, however, isn't fully understood. Prescription drugs are more likely to cause sleepwalking and night terrors, particularly in older people on medications for heart disease. In young and middle-aged adults, psychological factors may play a role in chronic cases, especially among victims of childhood sexual abuse and patients suffering from post–traumatic stress disorder. At the Stanford University Sleep Disorders Clinic, somnambulism and night terrors are so prevalent among Vietnam vets as to account for a clearly identifiable subgroup of parasomniacs— what one might call the sleepwalking war-wounded. In home settings, parents often report that sleepwalking is more common on nights when their child is overtired. It may be a sign of emotional problems or only of an urge to pee, yet most often the precise etiology in children remains unknown.

Having never seen a sleepwalker myself, I look into the feasibility of observing one at a sleep laboratory. Apparently, though, it's quite unusual to witness somnambulism in a clinical setting. Strange surroundings suppress such behavior. In any case, movement would be inhibited by the attached electrodes and confined space of a laboratory. It occurs to me that Dr. Kleitman may never have seen a somnambulist in his whole career. Now, I am really intrigued. I am just as curious to know why some of us *stop* walking in our sleep as I am to know why we start. I determine to find out.

I place an ad in the *New York Times*. Casting a broad net for any parasomniacs or insomniacs out there, I ask people to write and tell me their stories. On the third day, the first letter appears: "I have a sleep disorder, whereby if I eat a large quantity of carbohydrates I feel sleepy [for] approximately twenty-four hours from the time of that meal," a gentleman named Wallace writes from Long Island. "My bowels become constipated, and only after a bowel movement, will I begin to feel better."

Oh, dear. I'm afraid that I've run a personals ad for the deeply sleep-disturbed.

Each day for several weeks, I receive one or two more letters. They look identical, arriving in the same generic white envelope with the same flag stamp. The first sleepwalker to write is Judith, twenty-eight years old, one of those exotic birds who has been sleepwalking regularly since she was a little girl. In fact, I realize, it could have started much earlier than she thinks, before she was even able to stand up. Although it usually goes undetected, some babies have a parasomnia called confusional arousals, in which they move about in their cribs. It may begin with simple actions—sitting up while asleep, picking at the blankets—and over time progress to complex behavior. It's even possible that a toddler's first steps are taken as a budding somnambulist.

As a child, Judith writes, she'd often sleepwalk into other family members' rooms and climb into bed with them. Once, at summer camp as a ten-year-old, she sleepwalked to a neighboring cabin, where she woke up the next morning—in the bunk bed of another girl. Whether this tendency has also continued into adulthood, she doesn't say, yet I can't help thinking that her sleepwalking is rooted in a primitive human desire: homesickness for another body, its warmth and company in the dark.

"Are you interested in bilingual sleepwalkers?" asks Virginia, a middle-aged woman from Connecticut. In a long letter, she confides that her husband has the amazing ability to sleepwalk while speaking in both Arabic and English. Raised in the United States by immigrant parents, with Arabic as his first language, her husband hadn't used this tongue since early childhood; in wakefulness, he can hardly recall a word. Sleepwalking is rare in adults, but to also be a fluent bilingual sleeptalker makes him doubly blessed, like an ambidextrous person able to produce mirror-writing.

One startling incident took place twenty-eight years ago, Virginia continues, when their first child was born. They brought the baby boy home from the hospital, tucked him into a bassinet, and fell asleep. During the night, she woke to find her husband fussing with the baby. Her husband didn't respond to her when repeatedly asked what was wrong; he murmured in Arabic to the baby. Finally, he returned to bed. With morning, Virginia was shocked to find the boy had been neatly wrapped up in one of her husband's white, button-down shirts in lieu of a blanket. Although he remembered nothing at first, she prompted his memory by reconstructing the words he'd used. He eventually recalled having a nightmare in which the boy was endangered by the devil. The murmurings were a traditional Arabic prayer; the whiteness of the shirt was apparently meant to protect the baby. In his sleep, it seems, her husband had performed an impromptu exorcism.

Harriet, an elderly woman from Alabama, writes that one summer night sixty years ago, her younger sister, Betty, sleepwalked from the bedroom they shared to a second-floor balcony and dove off. It's no wonder Harriet can still hear the horrible thud as Betty hit the ground; she just missed a square of concrete, landing on grass, which saved her life. The girl had dreamt she'd been swimming. It reminds me of an actual case of "sleep-swimming," recorded by Dr. MacNish more than 150 years ago. "About two o'clock in the morning," he noted, in a town on the coast of Ireland, "the watchmen on the quay were much surprised at descrying a man disporting himself in the water, about a hundred yards from the shore." He had swum a mile and a half when a boat crew finally picked him up, "but strange to say, he had no idea whatever of his perilous situation: and it was with the utmost difficulty they could persuade him he was not still in bed."

During the Victorian era, one didn't need to sleep-*swim* to attract attention. Even the most mundane episodes of somnambulism (or noctambulism, as it was also called) were regarded with fear and astonishment. In sleepwalking, as in the hypnagogic state and hypnotic trance, the layers of civilizing influence were brushed aside and the "true volitional self" was thought to emerge. As Daniel Hack Tuke wrote in his 1884 treatise on the topic, in sleepwalking "the will is the slave of a dream or a suggestion."

Helpless against these forces, one might be driven to do terrible things while sleepwalking. Medical literature of the time is studded with sensational crime stories, invariably involving family members gone bad, such as that of the Scottish homicidal somnambulist Simon Fraser, whose case was described in an 1878 issue of the *Journal of Mental Science*. "The fatal occurrence was simple and tragic," D. Yellowlees, M.D., physician-superintendent at Glasgow Royal Asylum, wrote in his remarkably sympathetic account. "On the night of April 9th the accused was asleep in bed with his wife and their only child, a boy of about 18 months, of whom he was passionately fond. About 1 A.M. he saw a wild beast of some kind rise up through the floor and jump on the bed to attack his child. He seized the animal and dashed it against the wall or floor to destroy it. His wife's screams recalled him to himself, and he found to his horror that he had seized and fatally injured his child."

Fraser, twenty-eight years old, was a "tall, pale, dejected-looking man," Dr. Yellowlees wrote, whose "chief outward peculiarity" was his hair, which was black and stood "rigidly erect." Otherwise healthy, Fraser had been plagued by restless sleep and episodes of somnambulism, his father testified, since he was a small boy. More telling, his mother, maternal grandfather, and brother had all died from epilepsy, and his aunt and cousin were both inmates of insane asylums. Was Simon Fraser also insane and suffering delusions, one must wonder, or perhaps an epileptic in the midst of an unusual violent seizure? His trial was held in Edinburgh on July 15, 1878. On being asked to plead, Fraser declared, "I am guilty in my sleep, but not guilty in my senses."

He was found innocent of infanticide, "which he committed by reason of a condition arising from somnambulism," the court ruled. Set free, he was nonetheless sentenced to a form of solitary confinement: to sleep in a separate room for the rest of his life, apart from any other person.

Such vivid stories are difficult to reconcile with an irrefutable scientific fact: sleepwalking does not occur during REM, when most dreams take place. In fact, a condition of REM sleep—temporary paralysis of the limbs—makes sleepwalking in this state a physiological impossibility. Instead, it occurs only during the deep non-REM sleep of stages 3 or 4, when dreams are rare and waking is least likely. In my mind, this makes somnambulism far more mysterious. I've now got my own theory: a dream may first plant the idea to sleepwalk, like a scene to be acted out in a game of charades, or it may be the narrative imposed later to make sense of seemingly irrational behavior.

Roger J. Broughton, a Canadian scientist who coined the term *disorders of arousal,* has a different hypothesis. In a 1968 paper in the journal *Science,* he offered a provocative explanation for the paradox of sleepwalking with concurrent dreams. Pointing out that up to 15 percent of dreams are linked to non-REM sleep (stages 3 and 4), he thought these could be "dreams" of a distinct, not yet understood type. It is conceivable, he speculated, that in the deepest stages of sleep, "when the risk of subsequent recall is minimal, protective barriers are lowered" and a person's repressed "emotional conflicts" might be expressed in "mental activity" that could lead to sleepwalking. He noted that this non-REM mental activity lacks the hallucinatory story-lines of typical REM-state dreams. He likened it more to thinking than to dreaming, as different as words are to pictures. I wonder if this capacity might be enhanced in sleepwalkers—one leaves bed to act upon a thought, a burning impulse, even buried rage.

In 1987, Kenneth Parks, a twenty-three-year-old Toronto man, drove fourteen miles in the middle of the night, stabbed his mother-in-law to death, and strangled his father-in-law unconscious, all while sleepwalking, his attorneys contended. Parks did not fully awaken, they claimed, until he was back behind the wheel and found himself clutching a bloody knife. Horrified, he went straight to a police station: "I think I have killed some people . . . my hands," he muttered. In pretrial examinations, Roger Broughton and other doctors established that Parks had a history of parasomnias, all of which ran in his family: a chronic sleepwalker and sleeptalker since childhood (when he'd been a "severe bedwetter"), he also suffered night terrors as an adult. Even while incarcerated, Parks acted strangely in his sleep—sitting up in bed with eyes open, mumbling—two cell mates reported. He had no recall of the murder, had no apparent motive for committing it, and showed what was viewed to be true remorse. Serving as an expert witness, Dr. Broughton testified on Parks's behalf that he likely committed homicide while sleepwalking. He was acquitted of all charges in a Canadian court.

A mild-mannered Arizona man, on trial for killing his wife in 1997, recently made the exact same claim of homicidal somnambulism. Scott Falater, a Mormon and a father of two, didn't deny stabbing his wife forty-four times as she screamed, dragging her body to their backyard swimming pool, then holding her head underwater (a neighbor watched him do it from his backyard fence), but he did deny doing it consciously. "He did it because he was sleepwalking," Falater's lawyer told jurors, though he did not have an extensive history of parasomnias. He was still asleep, the defense claimed, even when he ordered the family dog to lie down, washed his hands, and stashed the knife and bloody clothes in a Tupperware container found hidden in his Volvo. If, up to this point, his defense was holding together in the minds of the jury, it may have all fallen apart with a key prosecution witness. A coworker of Falater's testified that the accused had specifically mentioned the Kenneth Parks case a week prior to Falater's wife's death. In June 1999, the jury convicted Falater of first-degree murder; he was later sentenced to life in prison.

I'm not inclined to believe either of them, Parks or Falater. Still, I've no doubt there are instances of sleep-related violence during parasomnias. A small percentage of sleepers seriously injure themselves and others during night terrors, for example. Night terrors are not nightmares. They differ in three primary ways: night terrors occur during non-REM sleep, when movement isn't inhibited; they are not associated with vivid dream imagery; and the episodes are usually not recalled upon awakening. Among the letters I received is one from a fifty-nine-year-old man, Randall, who has walked in his sleep and had night terrors his whole life. In a macabre personal journal charting episodes over the past thirty years, excerpts from which he sent me, he describes a typical brutal night:

August 26, 1995: "Terror. 11:45 P.M. After an hour of sleep, sprained wrist, left knuckle skinned from punching wall. Collapsed and cried in the front hall."

While fleeing from and fighting back night terrors, Randall has destroyed furniture; injured the cornea of his eye; and repeatedly hit his wife, Tina, in the face, punched her in the stomach, and dragged her from bed, leaving her black-and-blue. It sounds like spousal abuse, but, Randall states, evaluation at a medical clinic has confirmed that this behavior occurs when he is asleep, and that he has no memory of it. Medical help could not save his marriage, however. On May 14, 1997, he made this entry: "Tina told me tonight she is leaving me. Some people don't survive this. I wonder if I will?"

Randall's case is extreme. Most people with night terrors don't injure others, experts say. Those who do might be suffering from an altogether different parasomnia, one not identified until 1986, REM behavior disorder (RBD). In RBD, the REM state itself is disabled—a neurological aberration allows muscle activity to continue functioning when it should not. Drug treatment exists, thankfully, that's effective in 90 percent of RBD cases, most of which are in older men. Left undiagnosed and untreated, it would be, I imagine, like sleepwalking in hell: people are doomed to act out their worst nightmares.

It bears reiterating that diagnoses such as RBD could not be made, nor the finer points of sleepwalking and night terrors understood, if not for Eugene Aserinsky's identification of rapid eye movement sleep. And his breakthrough in 1951 might never have been made without his eight-year-old son, Armond. I began wondering if the original REM sleeper remembers those nights from his childhood, so I decided to track him down.

My telephone call finds Dr. Armond Aserinsky at home in Pennsylvania, where he is a clinical psychologist, married, fifty-five years old. Our conversation takes place in November 1998, three months after Eugene Aserinsky died, at seventy-seven, when his car hit a tree near his home in San Diego—an unexplained accident, possibly caused by falling asleep at the wheel. The question of his father's legacy is, understandably, on Armond's mind; he addresses it directly: "One does not make a landmark discovery more than once in one's life, if at all," he says in regard to his father. "He went to his grave feeling that he had been improperly acknowledged for his contribution; that this had been stolen from him by Nathaniel Kleitman."

Armond speaks with both cool precision and warmth, a tone unique to therapists, as if he's recounting a long-term patient's case history. When his father earned his doctorate in 1953, he was flat broke, with a wife and two kids to support, Armond explains; there was no job offer from Dr. Kleitman and the University of Chicago. He took the only work he could find, a low-level job at the Bureau of Fisheries in Seattle, knowing that he'd left behind his "wonderful discovery." He eventually moved on to good teaching positions at schools in Philadelphia and West Virginia, yet he never resumed high-visibility research as a scientist. "He was a bitter and disappointed man," Armond admits. "His career should have been a brilliant one; he was a brilliant man. But it didn't go that way."

Listening to his voice, I picture Armond resembling Eugene Aserinsky as he appears in journal photographs from the 1950s: a short, compact man, fastidiously dressed in a suit and bow tie, with dark hair and a pencil-thin mustache; the face of Peter Sellers as Inspector Clouseau. Although they were estranged in later years, Armond recalls with fondness being part of his father's research as a little boy. It took place at night in the old physiology building at the University of Chicago, a drafty, stone-walled laboratory that looked like the set of *The Bride of Frankenstein,* cluttered with brass instruments and vacuum tubes.

"I slept for him a couple of times," Armond tells me.

"This was back in the days of rather primitive electrodes, so there was a long period of preparation." First, his father had to scrub Armond's skin with rubbing alcohol to remove any oil. The electrodes were dime-sized, cup-shaped disks, on which Eugene smeared a gritty electrolyte paste; he stuck them onto Armond's eyelids, ears, temples, and shoulders and secured them with paraffin and surgical tape. Finally, with a pneumograph bound to his chest to measure respiration and his hands strapped down, he looked ready to play his part: an exhausted little Gulliver with the wiry-haired head of Medusa.

"The big concern for me was going to the toilet," Armond says with a laugh. "What an ordeal it was for him to detach me! Picture these long wires coming out of the electrodes, attached to a little box. The first time, we walked down to the men's room with him trailing me with the box and wires. Subsequently, he improvised with a jar."

Armond remembers the mood of these nights with great clarity: "It was *work,* and I wanted very much to please him. It was a way I could play a role in something very important. I knew he was very smart, and he was excited about what he was doing. It's hard to convey, but I was very much aware of a scientific process—a process of discovery—going on. Very much a sense of 'Aha!'

"It was just the two of us," Armond adds. When it came time to sleep, "he was in one room with the equipment and I was in the other." What a powerful image: father and son, each alone and yet together, attached as if by a dozen umbilical cords; scientist and subject, wired by the filament of dreams.

While the test sessions were never frightening, Armond admits he was nervous the first night. How much would his dad be able to record? Could he secretly read his son's mind with the machinery? But after that first session, once Armond saw the ink tracings of his brain activity and eye movements and his father explained what it all meant, he understood the arrangement: It was *he* who held the secret powers. He remembers his father waking him up throughout each night, peering at him: "Armond, Armond," he'd whisper. "Were you sleeping? Did you dream? What did you see?"

I find myself taken back by memories, to age eight and a time when I, too, became a subject of intense interest to my dad. Now in the second grade, I'd reached some invisible milestone in his eyes; evidently, I was ready to be groomed by him. I might be playing with my sisters when he'd call me into his basement office on Sunday afternoons, the fall and winter of 1969 and 1970. It was a wood-paneled corner space, dominated by a large, green steel desk, which had been his father's. My sisters and I wouldn't normally wander in there, except to use the area under his desk or the closet (where he stored rifles and camping equipment) for games of hide-and-seek.

While his office didn't have a door—opening onto the larger rec room—it was clearly my father's domain, a place where he paid the bills, made long-distance phone calls, and read the paper in a black reclining chair. One wall was lined with books—biographies of Eisenhower, Patton, Henry Luce, Hemingway, Kennedy. The top shelf displayed helmets from his military career, including the shiny black, plumed helmet, like something out of Dr. Seuss, that he'd worn with dress grays at West Point.

Here, he would teach me how to be a gentleman. Using his heavy oak desk chair, he showed me the proper way to pull out a chair for Mom and my sisters: "Pull it back from the table, turn it to the side, so she can slide in, then tap it behind her knees as she sits down." The closet doubled as a car door to demonstrate opening one for a woman, pulling it with you as you stepped back. Every Sunday, we practiced tying a necktie, shining shoes, or shaking hands. I learned to step into a handshake, grasp the other man's right hand firmly, release it quickly, never looking at the hand itself; "Look me in the eye, Billy! Look me in the eye!" He once tried teaching me how to defend myself in a fight—a little shadowboxing. "Come on, Billy, put your dukes up!" I ducked and balked as my father sparred, but I'm sure our match wasn't much fun for him either. He quickly called it quits.

Once the tutorial was finished, we'd go on outings, he and I alone—to the rodeo, a hockey or baseball game, the horse races, the boat show. We might drive out to Fairchild Air Force Base, on the outskirts of town, to look at the fighter jets. I appreciate his effort far more now than I did then, when I acted as wary as if I'd taken a ride from a stranger. On the way home, he sometimes needed to stop by the office. The Coke plant, closed on Sundays, was quiet and empty. While Dad worked at his desk, I'd take a bottle of pop from his cooler and wander down the hall back to the warehouse, a large, dank space where Coke trucks were parked. The concrete was often still wet from the previous night's hose-down; the only light came from a few dirty windows. Cases of pop stood in towering stacks, dangerously high. One could happily get lost in there. Disappear. I'd sit down on an empty pallet and sip my Coke, fiddle with the bottle top. Squinted eyes turned the crate towers into a dark, underground kingdom. "Billy? Billy!" There's Dad's voice in the hall, muffled, as if from the mouth of a cave. "Billy? Billy?" I can barely hear him.

⤦

It's true that a sleepwalker should not be awakened. People used to think doing so could cause instant death, because it was so traumatizing to wake up in a different place from where one had lain down. Dr. MacNish claimed to know of many such fatalities, even among somnambulists with "strong nerves," which is why he and other nineteenth-century physicians recommended ways to curb the behavior. Marie de Manacéine advised placing tubs of cold water around the bed, to stop sleepwalking before it could start, but as Dr. MacNish pointed out, this in itself could be so startling as to cause heart failure. Others added that somnambulists were wily enough to step over the tubs. Daniel Hack Tuke wrote that admonishing a youngster before bed—telling him he *must not* sleepwalk—had proved successful. Not to be outdone, Dr. MacNish suggested tying a leash from the bedpost to the sleepwalker's wrist or, better yet, having a second person sleep alongside the somnambulist. And if, in spite of these precautions, one still walked in his sleep, he should be "conducted [back] to bed without being awakened at all."

Today, more than a hundred years later, Dr. MacNish's last piece of advice remains the soundest. While it's not life-threatening by any means, waking a sleepwalker will leave the person confused and disoriented. It's best to let the sleepwalker be. Of course, some safety measures are prudent. Move a chronic walker's bedroom to the ground floor, if possible; remove dangerous items from easy reach; install thick drapes over glass windows; and so on. In nearly all cases among children, however, the parasomnia will pass. Most kids outgrow it, as I did by age ten, with its cause left unknown.

One of the few things experts can now say with certainty about sleepwalking is that it often runs in families. A recent British study found that it is 45 percent more common in children when one parent was a childhood sleepwalker, and 60 percent when both were. Evidence for a genetic link is further supported by a study of twins, in which sleepwalking was found to be six times more likely in pairs of identical twins than in fraternal twins.

Dr. Kleitman first observed that sleepwalking may be hereditary in the 1939 edition of *Sleep and Wakefulness*. By way of example, he told a story that he'd learned from a French scientist named Clerici about a married couple and their four children, all of whom were afflicted with somnambulism: "One night the entire family arose about three in the morning, gathered in the servants' hall around the tea table; one of the children in moving about upset a chair. Only then did they awaken."

And what, I would love to know, did they say to one another?

Perhaps they were neither embarrassed nor confused, but elated: *"Yes, yes, at last we did it!"* They'd share a bottle of champagne and a toast: *"To us."* Their synchronized sleepwalking was a fulfillment of a kindred dream. A triumph of like-mindedness.

It's kind of a stretch to imagine my own family perfecting this strange ability: all eight of us waking at once around the kitchen table in a woozy state of postsomnambulism, each holding a bottle of Coca-Cola. Actually, I like the facts as I know them. Neither of my parents walked in their sleep, nor did my sisters. My sleepwalking was a solo performance.

I am still tempted to see sleepwalking as a dramatic plot device; it was used to such dazzling effect in *Lady Macbeth, Tess of the D'Urbervilles,* and other works that have captured my imagination. But, I must admit, its function in my life was ordinary. In spite of my Cheeveresque fantasies, I don't think it was a genuine desire to leave home, to escape, although I was, in fact, teetering on a fence at that age. Like a lot of kids in between childhood and adolescence, I was growing unsure of myself, of my role as the only boy, brother, and son.

That I did walk in my sleep says something undeniable about me and our home: deep down I felt comfortable there.

Sleepwalking is such an intimate act, and not without risks. I'm grateful that there was always someone to watch out for me at night, to steer me from harm. In this, I am convinced that I've found the reason most of us walk in our sleep, even if only one time, and it's marvelously simple. Why does the sleepwalker walk? To be led back to bed.

❧

Chapter 8

Sleeptalking

T HERE'S STILL the small matter of that gibberish to resolve. Shannon said I yelled and chattered while walking in my sleep. What was I trying to say? What couldn't keep till morning? My true intentions can never be known. For every word expressed in sleep, many more go unsaid, I would think. They are squelched, then forgotten, or lost when the alarm goes off.

The sleeptalker may never know the sound of this voice. One doesn't wake to or remember it; you hear *about* it. If you were to listen to a tape recording, you might not recognize yourself as the person speaking. Sleep-speech is the essence of unself-consciousness. It's often delivered at a raised volume. Although it breaks the silence of the middle of the night, this *un*self is in conversation with another. It is trying to make a point, asking to be heard. The scientific term for sleeptalking is *somniloquy,* a lovely word for this dissonant poetry.

Today's sleep scientists have almost nothing to say about somniloquy. For all the time they spend observing sleepers in laboratories throughout the world, they pay it little mind: a parasomnia "of no medical or psychological importance," current literature states. More research is now devoted to headbanging, which falls under the same technical classification as sleeptalking, "sleep-wake transition disorders." Both parasomnias usually occur early in stages 1 and 2, a lighter sleep than that found in sleepwalking or night terrors. Although somniloquy does also occur during REM sleep, there is no direct evidence that it dubs dialogue onto dreams. Its significance and frequency while sleepwalking are unknown.

Men and women sleeptalk, children and the elderly, even animals in their own way, yet scientific data on its prevalence is sketchy and highly variable. A small 1979 study estimated that 5 percent of the adult population of Los Angeles talk in their sleep, while an earlier survey conducted in London reported that 70 percent of adults do. It's unlikely that this discrepancy says something profound about the difference between the British and Californians; rather, it would seem to suggest nothing more than the unreliability of tracking adult somniloquy.

Young children, tucked into their beds, make a better research pool. They're usually asleep several hours before their parents, who are keenly tuned to their voices. A fascinating recent study in the Basque region of northern Spain, where both Spanish and Euskera are spoken, enlisted one thousand parents to listen closely and report on the sleeptalking of their bilingual children, 681 in all. Somniloquy occurred at least once a month in about half the kids, evenly divided between boys and girls, the researchers found. Most of them used their first language during sleep; a smaller fraction used only their second language—a finding that suggests to me that, for some people, unconscious emotional distress is best expressed in another tongue. Some things cannot be said any other way, just as a poem can't be translated into a foreign language without its original rhythm being lost.

In an 1897 letter to his friend Wilhelm Fliess, Sigmund Freud mentioned a bit of somniloquy uttered by his daughter. "Do you think that children's talk in their sleep belongs to their dreams?" he wrote. "Little Anna, aged one-and-a-half, had to fast for a day at Aussee, because she had been sick in the morning, which was attributed to eating strawberries. During the night she called out a whole menu in her sleep: 'Stwawbewwies, wild stwawbewwies, omblet, pudden!'" Freud later interpreted this as a typical wish-fulfillment dream, one of the first he cataloged, in which little Anna "avenged herself" for being deprived of something she loved. Beyond this instance, however, he published no extensive commentary on sleeptalking.

Up until the late 1970s, mental health experts considered sleeptalking a symptom of personality disorders, including "borderline schizophrenia, psychoneuroses, character neuroses, and overt homosexuality," as one textbook listed them. It became clear, though, that it was difficult to find a sane person who did *not* talk in his sleep. For now, the best that psychiatrists are able to offer is that "people under stress," young and old, are more likely to sleeptalk. I love that catchall phrase—it covers everyone I know. We are led to believe somniloquy is as natural as breathing. If you can speak and sleep, you may sleeptalk.

But it isn't that straightforward. There's a recent case on record of a sixty-eight-year-old stroke victim with aphasia (impaired speech) who is able to speak well *only* in his sleep. During somniloquy this man's speech is fluent and coherent, his neurologist reported—he tells stories from childhood. But this facility deteriorates upon awakening, when he struggles with every syllable. Conversely, some garrulous people never talk in their sleep. Why would this be? And why is one somniloquist more talkative than another? There's something awfully intriguing about a sleeper who bolts upright in bed and delivers a short monologue—granted, in nonsensical English, as if encrypted against prying, but a monologue nonetheless. My friend Amy does this regularly, according to her husband. I would sleep with them just to hear it.

I'd be even more pleased to spend the night with John, one of the few somniloquists who replied to my newspaper ad. This is a man with multiple sleep disorders, I learned when I spoke to him by phone. A single forty-four-year-old, prone to regular episodes of somnambulism, insomnia, and to "bedthrashing" so violent that his dog will no longer sleep on his bed, John had no idea that he also talked in his sleep until a girlfriend stayed overnight. That first time, she heard him sleeptalk for three hours without pause. But it was more than talking, she said the next morning; he was argumentative, speaking more forcefully than he did while awake.

John's long-windedness is rare. Dr. Kleitman described one case like it from 1933. It involved four girlfriends—all stenographers—who shared a large room at a boardinghouse. One of the women, Frances, who steadfastly refused to reveal a single detail of her new romance, began to talk about it one night ten minutes after she had fallen asleep. Although it sounded like one-half of a phone conversation, what an earful the roommates got! She didn't finish until two and a half hours later.

Frances apparently repeated every word she'd said to her boyfriend that day, as if her speech had been rewound and played again. John, on the other hand, seemed to be rehearsing what he would later say to a contractor working on his home—a confrontation about which he was anxious. The following day, John's girlfriend told him it had bothered her, though she never woke him. Had she been waiting for him to say something really interesting? John resumed his argument on the second night, with one change. Out of deference to her, it seems, he whispered in his sleep.

There's a theory that speech evolved among early humans, in part, as a way to communicate in darkness. Maybe somniloquy is a trace of that primitive development, bobbing to the surface from four hundred thousand years ago. Then as now, awake or asleep, speech originates in the same place, the voice box, lodged between the base of the tongue and the top of the trachea. It is composed of nine cartilages, each properly named: Cricoid, Thyroid, Cuneiform, and the rest, like minor Greek gods of language; these are connected by a constellation of ligaments and muscles. The voice box is not at all boxy. Triangular at the top, circular at the base, it is bottomless and lidless. Two pairs of vocal cords are stretched across this cavity. Opening and closing like eyelids, they produce raw sound when air passes through the trachea, causing the lower pair—the "true vocal cords"—to vibrate. Finally, sound is tooled into language with the jaw, mouth, lips, and tongue.

Of course, speech is not a purely physical process. It depends upon the workings of the mind. We cannot enunciate clearly without hearing words spoken and seeing them spelled (or feeling their spellings, as with braille), nor can we describe vividly without drawing upon sensory perceptions, memory, and the capacity to imagine. Could we talk in our sleep if we didn't sense or fear or desire something in our dreams?

❧

Some nights I lie in bed, resigned to sleeplessness, and listen for sleeptalk through the papery walls of our apartment building. Every once in a while a voice goes off, like a car alarm jostled by wind. There's Betsy, the old lady next door. She interrupts her snoring to utter a string of words, as if reading ingredients from a recipe card. Other nights, Steve murmurs beside me. He seems to be struggling to say something important. I pat his arm, tell him it's okay; he turns over, quiets down. Sometimes the couple's dog upstairs, Pooter, whimpers and barks, his tail thumping the rug, as if he's chasing away nightmares. This always awakens someone overhead. Feet find slippers and shuffle to the bathroom.

I used to hear our former downstairs neighbor's somniloquy, a sound made more plaintive by the knowledge that she lived by herself. It was babble through the floorboards, yet had its own internal rhythm. Someone eavesdropping through another wall might have guessed she wasn't sleeping alone, that maybe it was not her. And in truth, it really wasn't her—at least not the delicate, silent woman we passed in the hallway. Low and aggressive, it was the admonishing sound of a self she'd never see.

If I'd knelt to the floor and called out a question, I wonder, would she have heard me? Would she have answered?

In *The Philosophy of Sleep* (1834), Robert MacNish claimed that one could learn to "converse" with a sleeptalker and thereby "extract from him the most hidden secrets of his soul." In this manner, he reported, a gentleman learned of his wife's infidelity and that she'd arranged a liaison with her paramour for the next day. It sounds like a tale inspired by Lord Byron's 1816 poem "Parisina," which was said to be based on a true incident—an affair between an Italian nobleman's wife, Parisina, and Hugo, her stepson:

> *And Hugo is gone to his lonely bed,*
> *To covet there another's bride;*
> *But she must lay her conscious head*
> *A husband's trusting heart beside.*

But fever'd in her sleep she seems,
And red her cheek with troubled dreams,
And mutters she in her unrest
A name she dare not breathe by day,
And clasps her lord unto her breast
Which pants for one away.

The actual Parisina was beheaded for her adultery; the fate of Dr. MacNish's unfaithful sleeptalker was not divulged. MacNish did go on to tell other anecdotes—all secondhand, of course. He'd heard about an American who preached in her sleep, performing every part of the Presbyterian service, from the psalm to the blessing. This woman, "the daughter of respectable and even wealthy parents, . . . disturbed and annoyed her family by her nocturnal eloquence. Her unhappy parents, though at first surprised, and perhaps flattered by the exhibition in their family of so extraordinary a gift, were at last convinced that it was the result of disease." Seeking medical help, her parents brought her to New York and other major cities, where her sleeptalking became something of a sideshow curiosity.

"Ear-witnesses" had told Dr. MacNish that "it was customary, at tea parties in New York . . . to put the lady to bed in a room adjacent to the drawing-room, in order that the dilettanti might witness so extraordinary a phenomenon."

I have no such gift for somniloquy, according to Steve. He hears me say just an occasional word or two, a fact that I find a little disappointing. I'll never know for sure if I sleeptalked as a child, other than during that one episode of sleepwalking. After age eight, I had my own bedroom and always slept with the door closed. No one in my family remembers hearing anything unusual through the walls. But I bet that I did. And, assuming that we take our vocal quirks with us to bed, then I sleeptalked with a lisp—a minor defect that, by day, required sessions with Comstock Elementary's speech therapist.

I don't know who decided that my speech needed repair—my parents or a teacher or our family doctor, Gil Porter, who also happened to be the father of my best friend, Chris. In any case, I'm sure I didn't object. I might have brought it up myself. Although unable to enunciate the word *sissy*, I considered myself a walking, talking definition.

The therapist traveled throughout the school district, a combination of medicine man and Avon lady, dispensing remedies and moving on. She didn't have a name, at least not an easy, memorizable one. She was just The Speech Therapist, known for dressing nicer than any of the other teachers. I recall her matching black dress, beaded necklace, high heels, glasses, and purse. The Speech Therapist couldn't have been from Spokane. Like the itinerant Art Teacher, she must have come from California. Once a week when I was in second grade, she set up shop in a makeshift office, behind a partition, and all of us with speech impediments lined up. An audience to others' sessions, I knew, at least, that I was not as bad off as Peggy Reardon, a classmate with hearing aids who spoke as if she had too much tongue.

My sibilance had become more pronounced as my permanent front teeth grew in, separated by a gap that added to my voice a persistent whistle. The Speech Therapist had me recite sentences made of the very words I had most difficulty saying. This was like trying to cure a sweet tooth with candy, I thought. Why not practice sentences that I could actually *say* and avoid all others? Yet week after week, she held up a mirror and instructed me to bite down, tuck my tongue in, and repeat variations of *Sally sold seashells at the seashore.* After a few months, the whistling hole in my voice was sufficiently patched up and I returned to my regular classroom.

On my own, I continued practicing her lessons all through grade school. The attention she gave my voice prompted a fascination with it. I became verbally precocious but remained soft-spoken. Even after I reached junior high and my voice changed, its gentleness continued as an embarrassment. I worried that it would reveal darker truths, like a person who betrays his secrets while sleeptalking.

Where I grew up, men had loud, gruff voices. I remember Dr.—never Mrs.—Porter bellowing from their front lawn: "Chriiiiiiiiiissssssss!" We could hear it from Comstock Park's swimming pool, a block away. (Dr. Porter also had a talent for duck calls; he could single-handedly have changed migration patterns.) And Mr. Booth, one of the few male teachers at Cataldo Middle School, which I started attending in sixth grade, easily quieted an entire playground with his punishing roar. At home, reading in my room, I could hear my father's voice over those of his guests at my parents' weekly dinner parties. Dad was gregarious (as was his own father, I'm told), especially after two or three Scotch and sodas. He was no less talkative after the guests left and we kids emerged from our rooms. Overeager to micromanage the cleanup Mom always had well in hand, he was quick to give us instructions. Like my sisters, I was trained to obey his word, to speak only when spoken to.

I found another way to express myself. I began to write stories and poems, an ability that I've fancied was a literary adaptation, a mechanism for surviving the environment in which I grew up. This is just a writer's musings, however, with some backward wishful thinking. Not every trait bears a causal link, an evolutionary biologist would say. Not every bodily organ or physiological effect still has a reason for being. The appendix is a case in point. Wisdom teeth, another. So, too, perhaps is somniloquy.

If it serves an adaptive purpose, it is not to rouse the

sleeptalker, whose ears are proofed against the sound. Nor would sleeptalking have helped in prehistoric days if you were asleep in underbrush, fearful of predators with far better hearing. Sleep leaves us at our most vulnerable. You'd think that natural selection would have chosen against somniloquy, whereas, instead, it has ignored it. Perhaps then, sleeptalking remains the biological equivalent of a dripping faucet—a pointless, vocal leak that serves only to wake others up.

In the annals of sleep research, I found one man who needed no convincing of sleeptalking's value, a scientist whose fascination with it exceeded my own: Arthur M. Arkin. *Found* is a bit misleading: I came across his abbreviated name while skimming a bibliography. It was his initials, *A.M.*, that caught my eye (was it a pun?): while his subjects slept, he remained awake, devoting himself for more than twenty years, I later learned, to the study of somniloquy.

Born in New York City in 1921, Arthur Malcom Arkin began his freshman year as a University of Chicago science major in the fall of 1938—the same semester Nathaniel Kleitman resumed teaching duties there following his stay in Mammoth Cave. Whether or not their paths ever crossed in a classroom, I don't know, yet I'd bet the student was well aware of the celebrated physiology professor, whose summer cave-dwelling had made the national newspapers. I'd like to think that the young Arkin was inspired by Dr. Kleitman's bold experiment.

After graduating, Arkin earned a doctorate in psychiatry at New York Medical College, became a psychoanalyst in private practice, and taught at City College of New York. While he conducted a broad range of research and coedited a well-regarded academic text, *The Mind in Sleep* (1978), Dr. Arkin's greatest contribution to the field was his six-hundred-page book, *Sleep-Talking: Psychology and Psychophysiology* (1981), published shortly before his death.

His aim with the book was to collect under one cover every significant scientific writing on somniloquy. Arkin references Aristotle, Darwin, and Freud, yet the book focuses chiefly on findings since the midfifties, including his own. It remains the world's first, only, and probably last complete scholarly resource. In addition, the book's appendices contain verbatim transcripts of six hundred individual sleep-speeches—every groan, pause, and mumble—most of them taped in Arkin's laboratory, together with the sleepers' EEG recordings. Each snippet of speech is matched to the REM or non-REM stage and the period of sleep during which it was recorded, as well as to the subject's dream recollection and thoughts upon awakening.

Beyond cataloging specimens of somniloquy, Arkin used these tapes in his own research. His initial goal was to take psychoanalytic theory to the next level—to marry Kleitman and Freud, in a sense—to provide a new tool for therapists. We dream regularly, as Aserinsky and Kleitman proved, and yet we don't usually remember dreams well or for long. Sometimes we're left with nothing but vague impressions. With sleeptalking, Arkin thought he could go right to the source— open a window into the subconscious mind and get reports on dreams in progress. He wished "to eavesdrop on them," to "glimpse the phenomena nearly *naked*," he admitted, slyly acknowledging the erotic nature of some dreams, as well as the voyeurism implicit in scientific observation of human behavior. Furthermore, he desired nothing less than "gaining control over sleeptalking," an ambition akin to training a butterfly to walk.

Dr. Arkin's early attempts involved presleep hypnosis. The occurrence of a natural dream would be a posthypnotic signal for his research subjects to talk in their sleep and describe what they were seeing, much as a TV reporter gives on-the-spot commentary. "Needless to say," Arkin wrote, "results fell short of the ideal goal." Another experiment involved doping subjects with fifteen milligrams of dextroamphetamine spansule and one hundred milligrams of pentobarbital. They slept like a dream but failed to elaborate. In another laboratory, a colleague tried to produce somniloquy through escape-avoidance techniques. With this experiment, it was as if the butterfly had flown into a bug zapper. Night after night, he subjected three young men with no history of sleeptalking to continual noxious light and noise once they were asleep. Only if they talked would the unpleasantness cease.

At last, success! I can imagine Dr. Arkin's delight as he heard a somniloquized men's chorus of words and screams. Still, the positive results paled next to the sleep-speech of a man Arkin had met five years prior: Dion McGregor. An American sleeptalking savant, Dion (rhymes with *lion*; short for Dionysus) gained a few minutes of fame in the early sixties. His somniloquy was the subject of a 1964 book illustrated by Edward Gorey, *The Dream World of Dion McGregor,* and a concurrent record album of the same name, which has recently been released on CD with a new title, *Dion McGregor Dreams Again.* Dion's sleeptalking was uncommon in that it was so frequent, clear, and profuse. While some people suggested the recordings were a hoax, Dr. Arkin recognized them as "spectacular" examples of "macrodissociative sleep-utterance" —episodes lasting a minute or more. After interviewing Dion, Arkin wrote: "He impressed me as a sensitive, shy, honest, unconventional man with an artistic temperament, and certainly not psychotic."

Dion was forty-two years old when the book and the record were originally released, though at the time, he lied and said he was thirty-six. His author photo shows a pudgy, sandy-haired man with pockmarked skin, wearing black horn-rims. He brings to mind Billy Carter, Jimmy Carter's redneck, beer-drinking younger brother, until one hears his sleep-speech, that is.

"Ah, well . . . uh . . . don't look around. I know you can't see me."

On the CD he sounds as if he were channeling Truman Capote on acid: flirtatious, slushy, disconnected from reality— the voice of self-*un*consciousness. Even his transcribed speeches have this quality.

"There were four of us in that room," one speech begins. "We were just having a nice . . . we watched television a little while, then we decided to go out and get the Sunday paper. . . . We opened it up, each of us took a section, and disappeared."

Suddenly, his voice becomes agitated: "Oh, God, if you want to find me, look in the Book Section," Dion cries. "I disappeared into the Book Section. Yes. Jimmy vanished into Sports. Yeah, oh, it's just awful! Awful! Mike's in the Magazine Section. Yes, I don't. . . ."

Dion, who died in 1994, never understood the interest people took in his sleeptalking. As he once said, he couldn't take credit for *writing* the book or recording the album—they were composed of tapes of his sleeptalking, over which he had no control, and he recalled none of it. To him, it was like being famous for wetting the bed. He'd rather have been remembered for cowriting the song "Where Is the Wonder?" which appeared on Barbra Streisand's 1965 album, *My Name Is Barbra;* or for the one book he did write, *The Films of Greta Garbo.* But it wasn't to be; few people remember Dion the lyricist or Hollywood archivist. A somniloquist since age four, Dion developed into one with astonishing gifts. It might have gone undocumented had he not become a struggling songwriter, so poor that he had to sleep on his friend Michael's couch. Awakened almost every night by Dion's sleeptalking, Michael soon began recording it.

"How do we get out? How do we get out? How *do* we get out?" Dion's newspaper rant continues.

"Yes, the political page . . . just swallowed us up. No, it didn't hurt really. It felt sort of dusty and dry as we were pressed in. . . . I can talk to Skip from the Book Section; Mike can talk to Jimmy from Sports. . . . We can move. Yeah, we go from section to section. The entertainment page is fun. And some of the ads are nice. . . ."

Michael taped Dion for seven years, long after the book and record both failed to earn them any money. The only reason Dion allowed the taping to continue, he said, was because he hoped it might provide lyrics for a new song, maybe even another hit for Barbra.

"It's swinched, it's very swinched. Humph, now why? Anybody can swimble. But have you ever swinched? Yes, the world is swimbling. Ummmm. . . ."

But, sadly, no. Not even a B-side.

As Dr. Arkin noted, Dion's speeches sound as if he's chatting with imaginary companions who reply in kind, for there are appropriate silent pauses. This is typical of somniloquy, although the extent to which Dion carries on an "inner dialogue" is not. In most cases, sleep-speech is brief and composed of grunts, a few words, or unfinished sentences. Whether sleeptalkers can be engaged in dialogue is another matter. Bed partners often claim they've had talks with their sleeptalking mates, and Dr. Arkin was eager to document this in his lab. Despite his best efforts with bona fide somniloquists, however, he could not prove that meaningful conversations ever take place. When a person thought to be asleep responds to questions, Dr. Arkin supposed, he or she may actually be awake but very drowsy.

As to why humans sleeptalk, Dr. Arkin ultimately concluded that somniloquy reflects a concurrent "mental stream"—what one is *thinking* while one is sleeping. Although everyone has these thoughts, some people, sometimes, spontaneously verbalize them, while others never do. It may occur when the balance between sleep and wakefulness becomes unstable—perhaps for a few seconds you are in neither state. In the midst of this "lively psychophysiological fracas," Dr. Arkin theorized, somniloquy is formed.

"Oh, yes, tongues wag in this town!" Dion confides in another speech. "From the highest banker right down to the lowliest sweeper in the tradesman store. Tongues wag. . . . And they've got a lot to wag about. Hmmmph! Well, take old Mrs. Smith-Rhonson . . . *she's* got a secret. Yes! It's about her son."

In point of fact, people rarely give away secrets while sleeptalking, Dr. Arkin found. A person secretive by day will be secretive at night. Even Dion McGregor, a kind of sleeptalking exhibitionist, apparently never disclosed his most private thoughts or deeds, nor anyone else's, for that matter. On the contrary: his sleep-speech bore little relationship to his waking life. And while Dr. Arkin had originally hoped that somniloquy would provide insight into dreams as a tool for psychoanalysis, in practice it didn't. As Dion talked, for instance, it's doubtful he ever saw the surreal imagery he described. Dion himself confirmed this—his dreams and speeches rarely matched up. He didn't know *what* to make of what he said.

"He has *hands,* and *elbows,* and *arms,* and *no wrists!* She tries to hide this fact . . . I don't know . . . what's the secret behind Mrs. Smith-Rhonson's son's wrists?"

As innocuous as Dion's words sound today, I am still haunted by the possibility that a very troubled soul lay at the heart of this flamboyant man who talked in his sleep, whose somniloquy was recorded, published, exploited. Dressed up with Gorey's whimsical drawings, his book looks enchanting. On the written page, his sleeptalking references are often funny, campy, graphic, fantastical. But listening to the recordings, one finds that Dion's somniloquy nearly always ends in the same way: in fury, with a bloodcurdling shriek.

⟨≈⟩

Although Dion McGregor never sought a cure to end his sleeptalking, one arrived, by chance, in 1980. At age fifty-nine, he fell in love with a man named Clement Brace, with whom he remained until his death. After meeting his partner, Dion told others, his sleeptalking stopped.

The only other somniloquy cure I've heard about was one tested in Bermuda in the late 1970s by Dr. Alan Le Boeuf. A twenty-seven-year-old naval officer was seeking treatment for his sleeptalking because his girlfriend had become fed up with its frequency and volume. Prior to consulting the doctor, the patient had tried drug therapy and hypnosis, both with no success.

Dr. Le Boeuf used aversion therapy. At the onset of a talking episode, a one-hundred-decibel tone was automatically delivered through an earpiece, causing the sleeper to awaken. The man's first instinct was not to stop sleeptalking but (like John, the argumentative sleeptalker who wrote me) to talk more quietly. He, too, learned to whisper in his sleep. Circumventing this development, Dr. Le Boeuf taped a small microphone to the patient's throat, which caught every sound, prompting the tone to resume. By the end of treatment, somniloquy had ceased.

Current research indicates that people like Dion McGregor and the Bermudan man are genetically predisposed to somniloquy (as is also often the case with sleepwalking and insomnia). A 1984 study suggests that a single genetic factor causes both chronic sleeptalking and sleepwalking, and that sleeptalking is actually a milder manifestation of this disorder. One of the earliest reports I've found of the hereditary link in sleeptalking is from 1904. In the *Proceedings of the American Medico-Psychological Association,* Dr. Dwight R. Burrell described a patient identified as "D.," a thirty-two-year-old farmer, the eighth of ten children in a family of somniloquists. "The tendency apparently came from the paternal side," he wrote. D. "talked some as a child, more freely as a young man, and improved with years. . . . His conversation assumed a wider range, and was more like that of the waking state."

Of the many sleeptalking incidents Dr. Burrell described, the most fabulous involved D. and a brother who had returned home after two years away. The siblings shared a bed that first night and, according to "ear-witnesses," got reacquainted through sleeptalking: "While sleeping together, they exchanged news, and rehearsed personal experiences, punctuating the same with snores and laughter. . . . Alas, it was a wasted visit," Dr. Burrell concluded, "for they recalled nothing whatever of the occurrence upon waking in the morning."

The story is charming yet hard to believe. Even so, D. and his brother have inspired me. If I talked in my sleep while growing up, then maybe my dad, mom, and sisters did as well. Perhaps we even spilled our secrets, though I know sleeptalkers seldom, if ever, do this. I can imagine each of us asleep in our bedrooms many years ago. I am thirteen years old. It's the middle of the night. Mom's snoring competes with my youngest sister Julia's. There's the sound of Dad grinding his teeth. Without rising from our beds or stepping from our dreamworlds, one at a time we say what we are privately thinking.

Ellen, the second eldest, describes how scary it is to have Hodgkin's disease, especially since her illness is never discussed. Lying very still by herself in the dark, she feels most sick. Shannon, who struggles to get C's in school, says she knows she's stupid and worthless. But can't someone take time to help her? Mom admits how exhausted she often is, caring for six children. And she weeps as she talks for the first time about her friend Linda, a mother of four who lived nearby and recently committed suicide. Each family member speaks—seven disembodied voices, behind closed doors—and then it's my turn.

I begin loudly, then stammer and stop. I start over. It's gibberish at first, then I finally get it out. I tell them I've been attracted to men since I was a boy. There's no response—not a question or an admonishment—just silence. So I continue telling my story. The walls of my room fold open into pale sky as I proceed. Before I can finish, it's morning. I pass my sisters in the hall and bathroom. Mom's still in bed. I glance at my father over breakfast. He mentions a poor night's sleep, nothing else. His jaw clicks as he eats his cereal.

Chapter 9

❧

Arousals

T HEY REMEMBER nothing. I finish breakfast, get dressed—blue cords, white shirt, red cardigan, the uniform of Cataldo Middle School. I sit through classes, barely breathing, and hide out in the library during lunch, half expecting to be hauled away to juvie hall. By dinnertime, though, I know for sure: nothing's changed, in spite of last night's disclosures, in this fantasy of my family. That is the beauty of sleeptalking. Unless another person's awake, listening, the words evaporate, like the last drop of water in the glass at bedside.

In reality, I didn't have the nerve to say my piece until ten years later, at age twenty-three. I felt sure I'd dropped many clues. Just in *being,* I was, I thought, homosexual. But, no. My parents, among others, said they never knew, never suspected a thing. It was not what I'd expected to hear. What they focused on was the reasons it could *not* be true (a series of girlfriends, for instance). They believed me in the role of a young straight man. This recognition was as troubling as my parents' distress: I had become so expert at *passing,* as they say, that I could render an essential part of myself unnoticeable.

Passing is perfected at a young age. It's a language of necessity, self-taught through inference: one learns how to improvise the stories by which to go undetected—first at home, then in school, at church, and outward in ever-widening circles; to create a *self* enclosed by ironic quotation marks. It left me with an indelible illusion of both control and passivity, of participating in life and remotely witnessing it.

When I came out, I was often asked, when did you first *know* you were gay? (A different question from, when did you become homosexual, or why are you one?) It was a polite way of asking, what the hell happened to you? *I always knew,* I'd say solemnly, *I always felt different,* in defense against possible holes in my alibi. It shut people up but wasn't true. I had no idea something was amiss until circumstances conspired in an innocent way, when I was eight years old.

I was in the TV room at my friend Drew Martin's house when his father walked in from a day of snow-skiing. Drew and I were sitting on the floor, playing a board game. While talking with us, Mr. Martin stripped off his sweater, his turtleneck, his T-shirt, his boots, two pair of socks, his ski pants. I registered every article of clothing as it dropped onto the floor. When I finally looked up, he stood above me, harmlessly, in his snug white thermal long underwear. He lit a cigar and sat down to watch TV. For a moment, I was transfixed by the plain sight of him, his stocky, hairless body, his trim mustache, the mixed scent of perspiration, fresh air, and tobacco. I wasn't conscious of a sexual impulse exactly. I simply knew that I, too, wanted to take off my clothes—a response not unlike that which I might feel around a half-naked man today. And I knew that my desire was shameful. This conflict between guilt and yearning was not only undiscussable, but unthinkable. Drew handed me the dice and I took my turn, playing the game as though nothing had happened, no rule had been broken.

It hardly seems coincidental that I began sleepwalking at the same age. The emerging facts of my life were causing little disturbances in my head. In a somnambulistic state, I sought out reassurance from my mom or dad, who would then put me back to bed. Such a reaction is not unique to one who happens to be homosexual. A variation of the story could be told by a straight man—say, Drew Martin—who as a boy perhaps glimpsed my mom in her slip through a half-opened door; who saw her for the first time as a body—breasts, nipples, creamy flesh; and couldn't quite get over it. Or by one of my sisters, had she been in that TV room, playing with Chrissy or Sarah Martin when their dad came in. But Mr. Martin most probably wouldn't have stripped down. In our presence, he felt comfortable because we were guys, like him.

His obliviousness and the naturalness of what he was doing, together with his athletic masculinity, made it all the more arousing. I'd seen men undress before—in a swimming-pool locker room, for instance—but it had never had an effect on me until that day. Something clicked.

Of course, my sleepwalking rationale is pure speculation. I never sleepwalked the five blocks over to Mr. Martin's house, and I seriously doubt I mentioned him in a bit of somniloquy. (To this day, however, I do have a fetish for men's long johns. Indeed, I sleep in them.) But then many things that we personally accept as "factual" have not been proved. That love at first sight is *real,* for instance. Or that there's life after death. To some of us, though, they sound right. They feel right. We take them on faith. So, too, the genetic origin of sexual orientation. There is no absolute scientific evidence for it, yet it makes intuitive sense to me that I was "born gay." By eight years old, I was ripe for a brief, startling homoerotic epiphany.

Which is not to say I understood sexuality. I didn't. But even a young child has a sensual awareness of his body; a comprehension of things that feel good, things that don't. Male babies regularly have erections, as Dr. Spock himself explained, and they play with their genitals, which may or may not be accompanied by a sense of pleasure. (They also play with their feet.) We don't really know. Nor do we know exactly why males have regular penile erections when we sleep, beginning as young as three weeks old.

William Alexander Hammond broached the topic in *Sleep and Its Derangements* (1869): "The erections which the generality of healthy men experience in the morning before rising from bed are . . . due to the fact that the recumbent posture favors the flow of blood to the penis and testicles." In addition, given that genital nerves arise from the lower spine, Dr. Hammond thought the penis was stimulated simply by lying on one's back, an act of frottage by association with a mattress. "Such erections," he hastened to reassure his readers, "are usually unaccompanied by venereal disease."

In fact, they may have nothing directly to do with sexual desire. A team of German scientists first formally noted the periodic cycle of erections during sleep in an obscure paper published in 1944. Eugene Aserinsky later filled in another crucial detail. In his unpublished 1953 doctoral thesis, he commented on the surprising coincidence of the timing and duration of penile erections and of the newly discovered REM state. Aserinsky suspected a connection. Nearly ten years later, scientists at New York's Mt. Sinai Hospital set out to test whether this was true. In laboratory experiments, they proved that nightly erections are synchronous with REM state onset, give or take a minute. The correlation is so close that an erection signals the arrival of REM sleep in men almost as surely as the burst of rapid eye movement itself. During eight hours of sleep, a healthy male can expect to have full penile erections for a total of one hundred minutes—about the same length of time he's in REM. Researchers have found a similar effect in women, in whom clitoral engorgement is also characteristic of the REM state.

As with many aspects of sleep, the purpose of nocturnal erections and clitoral engorgement is unclear. They may fulfill a periodic, physiological need to flush the tissue with blood and oxygen. They may also serve as test runs for the complex coordination of vascular, neurological, and hormonal systems each requires, much like a computer that's programmed to check its software and operating systems every time it's booted up. No matter how habitually a person may over- or underuse it while awake, the penis or clitoris still becomes erect about every ninety minutes during sleep. The same New York scientists who verified the synchronicity of penile erections and REM sleep in the early 1960s correctly postulated that the link is not erotic. As with clitoral engorgement, the nocturnal penile erection cycle is independent of recent sexual activity. One of their seventeen test subjects, "an overt homosexual," had regular nightly erections, they observed, in spite of his having had sex at least twice a day preceding each session. In a related finding, they uncovered no causal link between nocturnal erections and the sexual content of dreams, something that has since repeatedly been confirmed. In fact, relative to the number of dreams people have, sex dreams are infrequent.

It's surreal to imagine this cycle also happening while I'm awake: getting a full erection for no apparent, sexual reason; sustaining it for twenty minutes; and completely ignoring it while going about my daily business; especially with the knowledge that another erection will arrive shortly. It sounds like a writer's perfect distraction; I'd get nothing done. Yet, during sleep, both the male and female mind possess this level of ascetic discipline. The closest I come to imagining it is in recalling preadolescence, say eleven years old, when erections sprang at the unlikeliest moments, in class or church, like genital non sequiturs. In *Sexual Behavior in the Human Male* (1948), Alfred C. Kinsey wrote about this quirk, in which nonerotic stimuli can throw young boys into states of erection. His list of nearly a hundred possible erection cues, unintentionally hilarious, ranged from hearing the national anthem to finding money to seeing one's name in print.

By the time puberty hits at full force, there are no more non sequiturs. Sex is the context for everything. Medical texts talk of male adolescence as a transitional period with no absolute starting point, but I believe there is a defining moment that marks the threshold. It's something as dramatic and potentially mortifying—and as universal an experience—as a girl's first menstrual cycle. It's not body hair, which sprouts over many months, strand by strand, or erections, which have been around since infancy. The voice breaking is a good possibility. In my opinion, though, it's *got* to be the first wet dream, also called a nocturnal emission. One morning, you wake in a small puddle.

Your first horrified thought is that you've wet the bed, which seems appropriate, in retrospect: manhood arrives, and you feel utterly infantile. And then you remember your last dream, just moments ago. You finger the fluid on your pajamas and realize, at once, this is it: a vestige of the dream itself— sex, in all its warm milkiness—melted down.

For some young men, the first time is the last. Masturbation, if practiced frequently, can bring a quick end to wet dreams; it may preempt your ever having the first one. They're later usually replaced by having sex with partners, consigned to a pimply adolescence and perhaps forgotten. Yet I remain fascinated by wet dreams, in part because on occasion I do still have one. It's a fleeting physical sensation that can't easily be put into words. I spoke recently with an acquaintance who described his recurring night terrors as being "like a wet dream." Sensing my complete incomprehension of his simile, he explained how he can feel the terror mounting in his sleep, then there's a release once he screams, at which point he awakens in a cold sweat. To borrow and transpose his vivid analogy, then, a wet dream is like a night terror, involving sex rather than violence, pleasure rather than fear, and ending in a muffled climax rather than a bloody howl.

With regard to etiology, Dr. Hammond ventured an opinion in 1869: "It is probable that here again the position of the body conjoined with the heat of the bed has much to do in producing the erotic manifestations occasionally witnessed." Such occurrences might be prevented, he advised, by sleeping on one's side. As for Kinsey, he admitted that he didn't know why men have nocturnal emissions, but he enthusiastically recorded detailed statistics about their frequency. Nathaniel Kleitman was tight-lipped on the subject. In his writings, he never once brought it up.

Form follows function, a doctor today would likely explain: nocturnal emissions release built-up seminal fluid. This makes urological sense, but it's disappointingly reductive, lowering a wet dream to the level of a bowel movement. It fails to account for the *dream* in wet dreams—not a dream of sex, but sex in a dream—the psychic trigger for an involuntary orgasm.

The Roman poet Lucretius described this sensation with an amazing modern frankness more than two thousand years ago. Regarding older boys, he wrote in Book IV of his didactic poem "On the Nature of Things":

> *Once the seed*
> *Of manhood starts to fill their genitals,*
> *Beholding in their dreams a lovely face,*
> *A beautiful complexion, or a form*
> *Desirable and fair, are so aroused,*
> *So stirred, excited, swollen, that the deed*
> *Becomes reality, and a tidal flow*
> *Pours out to stain their garments.*

I've read of a funny, French euphemism for a wet dream, *faire une carte de France* (literally "make a map of France"), that manages to turn the splotch left behind into a vaguely patriotic gesture. But the humor may be lost on a twelve-year-old who's just made his first stab at cartography. What's the boy to do with these soiled bedclothes? And, upon finding them balled up at the bottom of the hamper, what's a mother to say? "He should be reassured—it is perfectly natural and is health-giving," advised Marie Carmichael Stopes, the trailblazing sexologist and bed-making enthusiast from the 1950s. The nocturnal emission "is nature's way of shielding him from the necessity to tie himself in matrimony before he is ready and has enough experience to recognize his life partner," she wrote in her book *Sleep*.

"Yet, centuries ago," she continued, wildly veering off on a tangent, "the power-seeking priests, rabidly anxious to create sin, made even this quite natural function into one. The attendant circumstances of confession, penances and a sense of guilt, all tended to increase the young man's natural difficulties in sleeping. Even today, echoes of this vilely false teaching travel round the by-ways and make many a young man needlessly anxious."

⎯⎯

I can't say that I did nothing to provoke my own anxieties about sex. Although it now seems foolhardy, at thirteen years old I began hiding pornography under my mattress. Or, what I viewed as pornography—magazine photos of Olympic swimmer Mark Spitz in a Speedo, seven gold medals hanging between his nipples, and of Michelangelo's *David*. I became bolder as I became desensitized and soon stashed explicit skin magazines that I'd bought at J. J. Newberry's. I was still quite catholic in my taste, buying both *Playboy* and *Playgirl*, as though keeping open the possibility of a latent bisexuality. But it was the naked men about whom I daydreamed. It's no wonder I had more and more difficulty in sleeping. When I turned out the lights, the fumes of guilt rose from the mattress like fresh printer's ink.

Good God! Under my mattress! It's a cliché out of a dumb caper movie, a place to hide the stolen loot. I suppose, subconsciously, it speaks to the powerful relationship we form with our beds that we want to *hide* things there—as if one's bed is an extension of one's body. But really now, did I think these clues would never be found? There was always a chance that Mom would change the sheets, that maybe she and the cleaning lady would flip the mattress. I'm sure that part of me wanted to get caught—to be confronted with it, punished, and then reformed, forever changed. It's not as if I didn't know I was sick. At Cataldo, a parochial school, we had religion class every day. The Church's teachings on homosexuality were clear to me, even though they were never expressly mentioned. As I interpreted it, certain things were so immoral they weren't talked about—a message that was reinforced at home, on TV, everywhere but in some books and magazines.

Perhaps my slight recklessness was hormonal—bad judgment as a result of testosterone. But I'd also developed a way

of romanticizing my transgression, of telling myself it was normal behavior—"a stage I was going through." Indeed, it *was*
the kind of thing almost every teenager does, male or female:
sneaking a peek at some flesh. I'd just conveniently forget at
times that my craving was a taboo one. A poor memory is the
best coping mechanism. I was surprisingly permissive of myself, fearless in my pursuit of small pleasures. One day I took
a bus downtown, crossed the Monroe Street Bridge to the
north side of Spokane, and walked a mile just to take a second, long, lingering look at a poster version of Burt Reynolds's
nude *Cosmopolitan* centerfold. I had glimpsed it in a store I'd
been to earlier with my mom and sisters. In a clacking rack in
the back corner, I found a smiling, hairy man on a leering
bearskin rug. I could scarcely hide my delight nor deny the
truth: I was a boy with the heart of a *Cosmo* girl.

The weird thing is, I never did get caught. If anyone had
come up beside me at the store, I could just as easily have
been staring at the facing poster of Farrah Fawcett-Majors. In
my bedroom, I always remembered to move the magazines on
cleaning days. I had backup excuses cooked up. I knew what
I'd say if the Newberry's cashier questioned me. I was prepared to be interrogated by the store's security guard or, for
that matter, by my parents. Of course, none of it was for me.
It was for this other kid, I'd have claimed—you wouldn't know
him.

I did have one close call when I was in eighth grade. I
had joined my parents on a trip, a not unusual circumstance (I
often got to travel with them, a privilege not always extended
to my sisters), although I don't recall where we'd gone. The
one thing that's stayed with me is the plane ride home. The
three of us were seated together, with me on the aisle. Shortly
after takeoff, I noticed a man opposite me, two rows up. He
was in a suit, dark hair, maybe forty years old. Throughout the
flight, he kept turning his head back toward me, glancing, like

a driver who wants to switch lanes but keeps changing his mind.

I knew what was going on. If nothing else, my fear told me; adrenaline pumped through my body with every heartbeat. I tried not to look at him. I would read two pages of my book, then look up. When I did, the man swung his head around. I'd read a full chapter, but he was always there, smiling kindly, patiently, when I finished. I didn't dare say anything to my parents. I smiled at him, my face flushed, radiant.

I suppose it's easy to think this was a pervert, preying on a young teenager. It doesn't make it more excusable to add that I looked considerably older than I was (I was already shaving and had almost reached the height and weight I am today), perhaps sixteen rather than thirteen years old. But the fact is, I was cruising him as fiercely as he was cruising me, without fully knowing the consequence of what I was doing.

When the plane landed in Spokane, he stood immediately and took a step toward me. I thought he'd lean into the row and tell my parents that I had been coming on to him. I was terrified. But Mom and Dad were talking and busily getting things together to disembark. I watched, breathless, as the man opened up the overhead bin right above me. He pulled out his suit bag, folded it over one arm, and dropped a small piece of paper into my lap.

It could have been an accident. If anyone had noticed, he could have said, "Oh, sorry about that," and I could have handed it back to him. Instead, he locked eyes with mine and nodded, as if agreeing with something I'd said. I snatched the paper from my lap, buried it in my fist. As he walked off the plane, I quickly opened it, without my parents noticing. On it he had written a name, a telephone number, and these words: *Call me.*

Without missing a beat, I folded the paper, put it in my pocket, and moved off the airplane. As my parents and I walked through the terminal, I saw him several steps before us. I had the sudden impression that this was a parade, not a disconnected crowd of people, and he was leading it. Everyone knows, I thought—my parents, the pilot and stewardesses who'd fallen into line, all these strangers, old people, kids: everyone knows you're a faggot. It wasn't a secret. The joke had been on me all along. I could hear people whispering as he led us through the terminal down a hallway with bright fluorescent lights. Wherever he was going, I was following. He stopped at the baggage carousel; my parents and I were positioned directly opposite him. He smiled. Like stomach acid, a taste of shame rose in my throat. At once, I broke away, telling my parents I was getting a drink of water, found a garbage can, and threw away his note. With it, all the voices went silent, the parade dispersed. When I returned to the baggage claim area, Mom and Dad were waiting with our luggage, and the man was gone.

For a while, I imagined that he lived in Spokane and would somehow find me, take me away, an idea that was either terribly romantic or frightening, depending upon my level of self-loathing. He was replaced by other male fantasy figures from my crinkly magazines. But they, too, didn't last. Every four months or so, I would enact a ritual purging and throw the pictures out, with a solemn vow to change my ways. But desire for men was always there, right beneath the surface. Masturbation actually did seem to keep it at bay. It turned homosexuality into a figment of my imagination, not a lifelong condition—a humiliating sign on my back that I could never remove.

Masturbation was another carnal sin, but I could receive absolute forgiveness for it every time I confessed it to Father Austen. (Thank goodness he never asked follow-up questions.) It was the lesser of two evils, something I obviously kept confined to the privacy of my bedroom. Not every teenager can do this. A strange, rare sleep disorder called Kleine-Levin syndrome principally afflicts adolescent males and is marked by intense sleepiness, great hunger, and indiscriminate public sexual behavior. When it strikes, it's as though the mechanisms keeping sloth, gluttony, and lust in check are out of whack. A mother who finds her overly sleepy yet otherwise well-behaved son masturbating in front of her Tupperware party may want to consult a specialist.

This disorder was identified in the late 1920s by two psychiatrists, Willi Kleine in Germany and Max Levin in Philadelphia. Levin's first case was a sixteen-year-old boy, "D.C.," who came under his care in July 1925. While typically "lively, athletic, and robust," D.C. was instead experiencing his third attack of "hypersomnolence" in a three-month period. The illness had begun with flulike symptoms, Levin reported in *The Archives of Neurology and Psychiatry*, and featured a bizarre fever-vision: one night, "while trying to fall asleep, he had seen 'glass bottles' floating around the room." After D.C.'s fever broke, he endured ten days of profound drowsiness. As this sleepiness subsided, his appetite then became ravenous. (Patients with Kleine-Levin syndrome are known to eat until they vomit, which does not stop them.) Discretion, I suspect, prevented Levin from explicitly describing the young man's sexual behavior. Finally, about three weeks after the first symptoms appeared, they vanished, and D.C. returned to his normal self. The second episode started two weeks later. The boy had a premonition that it was coming: as he told Dr. Levin, "I just felt consciousness leaving me."

This sounds like an apt description for one of the hormonal tidal waves of adolescence, the sensation that the ground is being swept out from under you, leaving you helpless to seductive impulses. The fascinating thing about Kleine-Levin syndrome is that it so greatly exaggerates aspects of male adolescence that we think of as commonplace. Many teenage boys are prone to odd eating habits ("pigging out," that is), sexual experimentation, unpredictable behavior. Sleeping patterns also shift dramatically beginning with puberty. The biological clock matures as surely as the sex organs: adolescents start going to bed later at night and waking up later in the morning. Like a chronic case of jet lag, it may take years to adjust to the time change. The teenage boy who sleeps until noon on the weekends is not necessarily lazy or rebellious, as a parent may think. In fact, recent legislation before Congress proposed that school days start two hours later in recognition of this biological development.

Kleine-Levin syndrome is most common and dramatic in boys, yet teenage girls comprise about one out of four cases. Although scientists cannot say with certainty what causes the illness, nor are there any effective treatments, leading specialists suspect a link to the hypothalamus, the tiny region of the brain that governs our drives to eat, sleep, and have sex. Hypothalamic dysfunction might be caused by a virus (which would explain the initial flu symptoms as well as the eventual recovery) or by an unspecified hormonal imbalance during puberty that leaves inhibitory functions damaged. Fortunately, episodes of Kleine-Levin syndrome gradually lessen in severity and frequency, then disappear altogether, as if they've been outgrown.

This same area of the brain has become the focus of a political and scientific debate about the basis of sexual orientation. In 1991, Simon LeVay, a neuroanatomist at the Salk Institute in La Jolla, California, reported finding a significant difference in the hypothalamus of adult gay and straight men. In postmortem examinations, a portion of the hypothalamus thought to be involved in regulating "male-typical sexual behavior" was, on average, two to three times smaller in the gay men, and about the same size as those from several women (none known to have been lesbian) also autopsied. Some thought at first that this was the Holy Grail of homosexuality, proof of nature over nurture, and a rebuke to all who claim that being gay is a choice (although LeVay himself never suggested this). But in reality the small study couldn't hold up under close scrutiny and LeVay's findings have never been replicated by others. This has left unanswered whether this brain difference was a cause of sexual orientation, a consequence of unrelated factors, or just a statistical fluke. The "homosexual hypothalamus" has ultimately been judged to be, at best, inconclusive evidence—one piece in a complex puzzle that may or may not also include a specific "gay gene."

Regardless of the science and the speculation, the theory still works beautifully as a metaphor for being homosexual. The hypothalamus is so small and deeply hidden, like a secret vault at the base of the brain, that it's unnoticeable to all except those who know precisely where to look for it.

⸺

I found my own indisputable proof on a family vacation in Mexico, when I was a junior in high school. Sitting with my parents and one sister on a beach in Mazatlán not far from the Playa Hotel, I couldn't help noticing a group of American men who had been in the same spot nearby for three days in a row. In their thirties, a little boisterous, drinking beer, laughing, these four men were not with any women. Nor were their swim trunks like those of every other man on the beach, including my father and me. Rather, they wore Speedos—purple, blue, red, green—as bright and shiny as polished glass in the sand. I could smell the coconut suntan oil gleaming from their hairless chests.

Every time I glanced over at them, one in particular always gazed back. By the third day, I had gained the nerve to test my self-discipline—and his attentions—just as I had a few years before on the airplane: I will wait ten minutes, then look up. There he was, smiling, eyes hidden behind sunglasses. I will see if I can go twenty minutes without looking at him. I couldn't. I will watch him for several minutes and see if my parents notice. They didn't. And when they left the beach early, my sister in tow, I chose to stay. When I looked up, the one in the inky blue Speedo placed a hand on the front of his swimsuit. He adjusted it suggestively, then waved at me.

All at once, I felt scared. I gathered up my things and began marching resolutely back down the beach to our hotel. Still testing myself, as well as him, I stopped after a short ways to see if he continued watching. Bending down to pick up a shell, I glanced behind. There he was, following me, as casual as a beachcomber. My limbs started shaking so hard, I had some trouble walking in the sand. Heart racing, overcome with nausea, I thought I might get sick. But I felt tremendously excited at the same time and wanted to take one more glimpse. I stopped to pick up another shell. Now he was even closer. When I stopped again, he was so close I could have spoken to him. In my soft voice, I could have told him to leave me alone. Finally, he was walking right next to me. He didn't say a word. His arm brushed against mine, then he walked ahead of me as I slowed down. We stopped at a deserted part of the beach in between hotels.

I said hello. The man in the blue Speedo crouched down and picked up a rock.

"You know, these rocks skip pretty well if you do it right," he said, tossing it with a snap to his wrist. The rock skipped perfectly in the surf—*plip, plip, plip, plosh*—and disappeared. "Here, you try."

"I've never been too good at that." I dropped the handful of shells and my belongings.

He picked up a rock from the wet sand, then inched up

behind me. "Let me show you." He put it in my palm, cupped his right hand over mine, and pressed his body against me, left arm around my abdomen. I could feel the warmth and slickness of his skin, and his penis against my lower back. I could smell beer, suntan oil, salty water. I flung the rock into the surf and it fell with a splash, then I reached back to feel him. "Yeah, something like that," he said, "something like that."

I stepped away. "I have to go swimming."

He followed me as I waded into the water. His voice glided as smoothly as the rock he'd tossed: "It's okay, this is okay. . . . You're very pretty, very handsome. . . . I've been watching you, admiring you. . . . I'd like you to come back to my hotel room. . . ." Soon, the water was up to our chests, waves pushing against us, and it seemed as if I were listening to him from underwater.

He said, "I'd like to touch you." He reached for my bathing suit and began tugging at it. "I'd like to kiss you." I couldn't say a word. "I want to make love to you." I wanted to ask him exactly what making love would include, but I was too nervous. If I open my mouth, I thought, I will drown. He looked at me intently, then his expression tightened, and he asked, "How old are you?"

My teeth were chattering. "Sixteen," I sputtered.

"Shit," he murmured, "I have a daughter your age." And you're old enough to be my father? I thought. I shook my head, so deeply disgusted with myself I couldn't think of what to say in response. He looked nervous now, yet didn't stop himself. Nor did I want him to. It felt marvelous, being touched by him. I had a jockstrap on, which he pulled down. I did the same, untying and pulling his bathing suit down to his knees. "You know, I used to always think it was wrong to get pleasure from another man's body or to come on to another guy," he said in his smooth voice. "But it isn't. It's perfectly

natural." He pulled me closer. Under the sun and clear blue
sky, the only thing obscuring us from view was a few feet of
water.

"So, when do you leave Mazatlán?" he asked.

"Tomorrow."

He looked surprised, then serious. "Well, we'd better get
back to that hotel room, now."

This is the part of the story I would turn over and over in
my head on sleepless nights for years afterward—erasing the
insistence from his voice, loosening his grip on my arms. And
all the while trying to give the encounter a different spin, a
fantasy ending in which he kissed and touched me with real
affection—to turn it into something it wasn't. *What would
have happened if . . . ?* I shudder to think, looking back on it
now.

I wanted to go with him but something held me back. I
stared at the empty beach, trying to figure out what to do. It
was as though I were watching the whole scene unfold from
outside of my body, from the perspective of a boy standing on
the shore, omniscient and unsparing.

"Come on," he urged. "Let's go."

It suddenly appeared, in every sense, wrong. I yanked up
my trunks. "I don't think so," I said, the words tinged with am-
bivalence. I waved him off and starting wading to shore, frustrated that I couldn't run, yet half hoping he would follow.

Chapter 10

❧

Blindness

WITH MY father at the wheel of our family car, driving seemed like an amusement-park ride when I was a child—part roller coaster, part bumper cars. Turning sharp corners and zooming down hills carried the thrill of veering out of control. He never got into a crash, thankfully, but our cars always bore the scars of countless minor accidents—dents and scratches, often incurred in parking lots, more frequently with cement posts than with other vehicles. The inside of our garage on Comstock Court looked as if it had been vandalized, its appearance in contrast to the extreme neatness within the house: fender-level gouges in the Sheetrock, bicycles left unridable by Dad's slight angling to the right while backing up. When I was in high school, the crumbling rear wall had to be entirely rebuilt. This history of vehicular bungs and mishaps could be traced back to Dad's being blind in his left eye and to the poor depth perception it caused.

The blindness was due to a detached retina, a combat injury. He had accommodated to the disability long before I was born and never liked talking about it with an inquisitive son. It didn't prevent Dad from playing handball and other sports. Nor did his eyes look different. I often couldn't remember as a kid which was the blind one. His "good eye" was the source of more morbid fascination. The notion that my father could lose his vision entirely—say, with one errant lawn dart or ski pole—was not hypothetical. His face was a moving target for my bad aim. If Dad went totally blind, the whole family went down.

In my conversations with Eugene Aserinsky's son, Armond, I learned that his father was also blind in one eye, the result of a childhood illness, and that we share similar memories. "It was never made clear to me exactly what caused the blindness," Armond confided. "I think that was due to the way he told the story. It was uncomfortable to him. He never clarified it."

I wondered if his father was ashamed of it. "The blindness itself was the shame," Armond responded, "not the method of getting it."

I was fascinated by Armond's disclosure, not simply because of the coincidence with my own father, but because of the irony: a half-blind man discovered rapid eye movement. And there was more. "He also taught at the Illinois College of Optometry while he was a graduate student," Armond added, "meaning that he had an expertise in the eye that predated his research into eye movement. He always said it was a happy accident—that Kleitman steered him in that direction. I don't believe so. This is a man who had an intense interest in the eye."

⮜⮞

Dr. Aserinsky openly acknowledged that his discovery of REM sleep and its relationship to dreaming was not without numerous precedents, historical and allegorical. "The prospect that these eye movements might be associated with dreaming did not arise as a lightning stroke of insight," he wrote in the *Journal of the History of Neurosciences* in 1996. One element already in place, he noted, was the work of L. W. Max, who had theorized in 1935 that people who dream would have simultaneous eye movement, although Max himself hadn't ever observed this. More important, the concept was deeply ingrained in popular literature, Dr. Asersinky wrote. "It was Edgar Allan Poe who anthropomorphized the raven, 'and his eyes have all the seeming of a demon's that is dreaming. . . .'"

The phenomenon was even alluded to in ancient Chinese history, as he pointed out. In a scientific paper published in 1948, two Shanghai ophthalmologists, Adalbert Fuchs and F. C. Wu, recounted the legend of General Chang Fei, who lived in the third century A.D. and reputedly slept with his eyes open. Although this must have made him seem like a terribly vigilant, invincible leader, it was probably due to a condition the doctors had observed in many Chinese people. It's called physiologic lagophthalmos or, simply, "sleep with half-open eyes."

Upon the death of a close ally, General Chang ordered a group of tailors to make three thousand mourning suits for his troops, according to the legend. The outfits were to be completed within three days, presumably to wear at the funeral. It was impossible to meet this deadline, but the general insisted: the garments would be finished or the tailors would pay with their lives. With death inevitable and nothing to lose, they conspired to kill him. One night, two tailors crept into his bedroom; their weapons, I imagine, were scissors. Hovering over him, ready to do the deed, they noticed with horror his open eyes rolling. Assuming he was awake, they turned to flee. On hearing snoring, however, and finding the general undisturbed by noise, they realized he was asleep. Chang Fei was stabbed to death, and his head delivered to his enemy.

Dr. Aserinsky cited the paper by doctors Fuchs and Wu in his 1953 *Science* article on REM. He was not quite so willing, however, to give unqualified credit to George T. Ladd, a Yale scientist who wrote in 1892 that he was "inclined to believe . . . that in somewhat vivid visual dreams . . . the eyeballs move gently in their sockets." Dr. Aserinsky was quick to point out the distinction between gentle movements and the rapid eye movements he'd documented. Ladd had made a good guess, in his view, not a scientific discovery. Similarly, he took issue with an assertion made by Edmund Jacobson, a physician who wrote in 1938: "When a person dreams . . . most often his eyes are active. . . . Awaken him . . . he will tell you whether or not he . . . has seen something in a dream." (Jacobson even claimed that these movements could be photographed as well as recorded electrophysiologically, though no such documentation exists.) Dr. Aserinsky felt certain that Jacobson and his predecessors, including the two murderous Chinese tailors, had in fact witnessed the slow eye movements of sleep onset. He had been the first to observe and record the unique, periodic state that he named REM.

Once he'd verified the REM state, Aserinsky began testing its relationship to dreaming. Although he strongly suspected the link, this had not been the hypothesis driving his previous experiments. One of his first test subjects was a blind undergraduate student whose eyes were capable of only limited motion. Aserinsky hoped to discern whether rapid eye movement itself is required for dreaming—that is, for "seeing" dream imagery. "On the appointed night I ushered the young man and his Seeing Eye dog through my recording room into a small sleeping chamber," Dr. Aserinsky recalled in the *Journal of the History of Neurosciences.* Once the electrodes and other devices were connected, he shut the door to the sleeping room and took his seat at the polysomnograph console.

At first, REM was indecipherable in the blind man. However, "I noticed at one point that the eye channels were a little more active than previously and that conceivably he was in a REM state. Since my usual criteria for recognizing REM no longer held, it was imperative that I examine his eyes directly while he slept. Very carefully I opened the door to the darkened sleeping chamber so as not to awaken the subject. Suddenly, there was a low menacing growl from near the bed followed by a general commotion which instantaneously reminded me that I had completely forgotten about the dog. By this time the animal took on the proportions of a wolf, and I immediately terminated the session, foreclosing any further exploration along this avenue."

Had he pursued it, Dr. Aserinsky would soon have discovered that blind people do dream, with or without moving eyes. Indeed, people *without* eyes dream. Moreover, neither the rapid eye movement for which REM is named nor the REM state itself is a requirement for dreaming. As noted earlier, up to 15 percent of dreams occur in non-REM stages.

The major difference between dreams of the blind and the sighted may be in their sensory form or complexity. In healthy adults with normal sight, all REM dreams are visual, a 1981 study concluded. In the participants' dream reports, the second most represented sense was hearing, at about 64 percent. Touch, taste, and smell all fell in at around 1 percent. Two additional sensations were tabulated: "temperature" was described in approximately 4 percent of dreams, and "vestibular" awareness in about 8 percent. Vestibular dreams are intriguing because they include activities that don't have waking-world correlates, such as flying, floating, and other surreal shifts in body position.

In individuals without the ability to see, the key criterion for having visual dreams is the length of time one had eyesight. For those blind from birth, visual dreams are said to be nonexistent. The experience may be primarily auditory rather than visual (rather like fetal dreams, as I've imagined them). For those who go blind at a young age, a visual component may continue for several years, only to gradually fade away, along with one's childhood memories of the experience of seeing. Adults who lose their eyesight may never stop dreaming visually. A friend's elderly mother-in-law, blind since her midthirties, still dreams of wildly colorful fields of flowers, for instance. Such individuals may draw upon a vast catalog of stored impressions, while also generating fresh imagery.

As explained to me by Ron Hideshima, a former artist who went blind twelve years ago at age twenty-five, one may lose the ability to see, but not to *visualize*. Now a computer technician at San Francisco's Rose Resnick Center for the Blind, Ron spoke with me over lunch. He said that he forms impressions of new people based mostly on their speech. One dazzling first impression came when he met his future wife, Kaori: "I envisioned a person with a wonderful, big smile." He soon dreamt of Kaori, though he'd never actually seen her. Her voice, in essence, was her appearance.

Ron took off his sunglasses before eating. His brown eyes were placid and immobile, but not without expression; his lightly scarred eyelids and brows punctuated his words. If there's little or no eye movement in the REM sleep of blind people such as Ron, whose eyes were ruptured in a major car accident, it may be because of damage to or degeneration of the eyes' nerves and muscles. It may also be because the movement isn't necessary; the quick scanning movement characteristic of REM sleep may be related to maintaining acute visual coordination—exercising the eyes when they're shut.

While blindness doesn't put an end to dreaming, it can

interfere with the ability to sleep well. Recent research confirms that 80 percent of blind people report serious sleep complaints, including chronic insomnia and daytime fatigue. This figure is at least twice as high as that for the general population. Some require sedatives to sleep and stimulants to stay alert.

Ron recalled a difficult adjustment in the first several months after he lost his sight, when he was confined to a hospital. "I would just doze off anytime. Since I had no visual perception at all, I didn't know if it was day or nighttime." Neither did his body. Without light cues, his biological clock was probably "free-running"—meaning that the circadian rhythms were unfixed, delayed about an hour each day—while also prompting his pineal gland to continually produce the hormone melatonin.

A minute level of eyesight may make a difference in establishing and maintaining twenty-four-hour rhythms; or, it may be that none at all is needed. Recent studies suggest that light signals travel from the eye to the brain along two separate ocular pathways: one for the light perception required for vision and the other for the "circadian pacemaker," the suprachiasmatic nucleus (SCN), situated in the hypothalamus. (The SCN orchestrates both alerting and sleep-inducing mechanisms, among other functions.) In some totally blind people, this second pathway may still work. The full extent to which light and darkness govern our lives, whether or not we can see, is becoming better understood. In my view, it seems as if we're wholly solar-powered beings, juiced up by the light of day and slowed down when night falls. I say *as if,* because it's likely not so simple.

The eyes may not be the only receptors for light cues. Researchers at Cornell University theorized that light exposure at the back of the knees could affect the biological clock. In their study of fifteen people, published in the spring 1998 issue of *Science,* they reported that circadian rhythms shifted as much as three hours following application of light behind the knees (a spot chosen for its distance from the eyes and for its ample surface vasculature). The results suggested that skin, the body's largest organ, may be capable of transmitting light signals to the blood, which then carries them to the SCN. Perhaps "skin-light" starts the wake-up process at daybreak before eyes open, it occurred to me as I read this report; it may even serve as a biological backup system, a way of supplementing the eyes and taking over in total blindness.

Two other research teams could not duplicate the results of the Cornell study, however, which has left the skin theory in doubt. In any case, darkness alone does not bring sleep any more than the sun makes us wake up. Interweaving factors contribute to the maintenance or disruption of sleep-wake patterns, such as social cues (work hours, scheduled meals), physiological effects (exercise, illness), psychological states (stress, calm), and technological developments—simple things we take for granted, such as air travel and the lightbulb.

After lunch, Ron and I walked the three blocks back to the Resnick Center. Using a white cane with his right hand, he held my elbow with his left. The force of his grip surprised me, as though he were pushing us forward in the direction he wished to go. It had been raining, and the wet streets made it hard to separate sounds, he said—they ricocheted like bullets zinging around in a cartoon. Sometimes a gust of wind swooped up sounds and carried them off.

Ron listened to his cane while simultaneously responding to my questions. Leaning in close, he told me that he'd only resumed a normal sleep schedule in his first year of blindness by enforcing a daily routine, and that it still takes a concerted effort, for which he is dependent on clocks. A "talking watch" is essential. When the sky isn't overcast, though, Ron can roughly tell the time and orient himself by the position of the sun. "If I feel the sun on my right ear, for instance, I figure it's about three o'clock—and I'm facing south." It struck me that, in addition to an acute sense of hearing, smell, taste, or touch, some blind people may have a heightened awareness of *time* that those of us with sight rarely possess; a sense of its capacity to impose order, to mark and carve out space. (Isn't the tapping of a cane like the ticking of a clock? Can't a minute be measured in footsteps? And, in passing cars, isn't the sound of time elapsing detectable?)

Ron's aluminum-tipped cane also yields tactile information, as if it's a long, unstubbable bare toe. "Through it, I can feel the street, curb, sidewalk, linoleum, et cetera," he said, "and it gives me enough leeway to take action—stop or swerve—if I do come to an obstacle." Of course, some hazards are unavoidable, such as reckless drivers. He and three blind friends were hit by a car several years ago. "I've learned that anywhere I go, there's danger out there. That's part of life."

After we said our good-byes, I watched as Ron nimbly crossed the sidewalk and entered the Rose Resnick building just before three skateboarders whooshed past. To be blind is to be alert to the unexpected, I thought to myself. The world of wakefulness presents risks, yet sleep can be a refuge. In dreams, a blind man may even see.

From my perspective, Eugene Aserinsky's path seemed predestined: his partial blindness led to an interest in the eye, which led to studying the eye in sleep, which linked him inextricably to the world's most distinguished sleep researcher, Nathaniel Kleitman. Which ultimately led to a bitter falling out, as inevitable as a son challenging the authority and beliefs of his father. With its rivalry, misunderstandings, and final betrayal, their relationship had a whiff of classical Greek drama.

Adding to this impression was a tragedy in Aserinsky's personal life, as his son Armond explained to me. Following the birth of a second child in 1952, his wife became seriously mentally ill and was institutionalized, at various points, as the family moved from Chicago to Seattle and, finally, to Philadelphia. In 1957, when Armond was fourteen years old, his mother committed suicide. He and his father never discussed it, and her death caused a rift between them, like a tree split by lightning. Through his teenage years, they became more and more estranged, Armond told me: "I was a reminder to him of very unpleasant times."

Still, father and son shared a passion for science. Dr. Aserinsky, who was on the faculty at Jefferson Medical College, secured some free lab space nearby to resume his sleep research. At age seventeen, Armond served as his assistant. It was reminiscent of the nights they had spent together at the grand University of Chicago laboratory almost a decade before, yet the sense of promise and excitement was gone. While Nobel laureates had seemed to haunt those hallways, Armond recollected, this spooky new building housed a ghost. The laboratory was located at the Eastern Pennsylvania Psychiatric Institute, where his mother had ended her life. "All the time, I was wondering in what exact space she killed herself."

A year or two later, when Armond was a college student, he helped his father in a REM sleep "demonstration" for a local television program. Once again, he was to be the designated sleeper. By his description, it was as if an old vaudeville team had been reunited for one last performance. The TV crew and polysomnograph equipment were set up in a surgical theater at the Psychiatric Institute, while a bed was placed in the adjoining glass-walled observation room. Once everything was arranged, the pressure was on. The program director reminded the Aserinskys that the crew was being paid double time, and they had just one night for filming.

Dr. Aserinsky said good-night to his son. "Hours passed with nary a sign of REM," Dr. Aserinsky later wrote in his 1996 article. "I began to worry. This was an on-location program already listed in the newspapers, a veritable crowd of TV people, nurses and other on-lookers were milling about in the confined quarters, and the production costs already were in the thousands of dollars."

About that time, Dr. Aserinsky continued, "I overheard one of the TV crew comment to the Program Director, 'Say, how will we know that . . . [he] isn't deliberately moving his eyes?' The Director responded, 'That's impossible, Mac. You can't move your eyes when your eyes are closed.' The cameraman shut his eyes and after a few moments of facial contortions answered, 'You're right.'"

No, he wasn't, Armond recalled with a laugh. He and his father had worked out a plan just in case Armond never fell asleep. "I'd practiced for some time beforehand doing simulated rapid eye movements. It wasn't easy! My father would give me a signal to do it, if necessary, when he'd come in to check the EEG leads. Neither of us had any ethical conflicts over it," he added. "This wasn't science, it was show biz!" Armond never did succeed in falling asleep, but with his father's clandestine bedside prodding, he gave Philadelphia TV viewers several flawless performances of REM.

I, too, had worked for my dad at age seventeen. He'd given me a summer job at the Coca-Cola plant after my junior year of high school. I was thankful for it; I'd be earning a union-scale wage. I couldn't make anywhere near that kind of money at Pizza Haven, where I'd been working as a busboy. At the same time, I was nervous. A year and a half after getting my driver's license, I found myself assigned to a delivery route and a six-

geared Coke truck. Up till then, my only experience behind
the wheel was in a Ford station wagon with automatic trans-
mission, power steering and brakes, and an eight-track tape
player on which I listened to nothing but Joni Mitchell.

I had to wake up at 5:45 A.M., a time I'd previously
known only as an altar boy. Now I dressed in the dark in a new
uniform: the gray-and-red, heavy cotton of a Coca-Cola deliv-
eryman. The year before, I'd moved into the basement bedroom, which my second eldest sister had left vacant when she
moved into a local college dormitory. It was, without question,
the grand prize of membership in our family—not only the
largest kid's bedroom in our house, but the only one with a toilet and shower. As the fifth of six, I was not the next sibling in
line to move in, yet as the boy I was granted special dispensa-
tion. I'd wasted little time laying claim to it, a zone free of purple Kotex boxes and electric hair curlers. The bedroom was
cool and musty, ridden with spiders, its wallpaper warped from
water seepage.

The room was so removed from the house's other inhabitants, it was like a secret fortress. It was far enough away, in
fact, to be effectively soundproofed. Who knew when your
music was too loud or Dad was demanding to see you? Which
was why my father rigged up a primitive buzzer whose wires
snaked from the bedroom, across the basement ceiling, up the
stairs, and to a little brown button next to the kitchen telephone. *Buzz* is too kind a word. It was reveille shortened to
one harsh note. Once Dad had his finger on the buzzer,
whether to go to church or come to supper, you couldn't possibly stay in the room. You had to run upstairs to escape it.

On my first morning of work at the Coke plant, I lay on
my bed at six-fifteen, dressed and ready to go and sick with
anxiety. I got down on my knees to pray for strength—a desperate last-minute appeal to myself, a private pep talk of sorts.
I'd secretly given up on Our Father's, Hail Mary's, and all the

rest several years before. Being an altar boy had not caused me to stop believing in God, but it didn't help. It certainly had not lessened my hatred of going to church. Nor had it enhanced my feelings toward my dad, who usually did readings at St. Augustine's 6:30 A.M. mass. Like all teenagers, I suppose, I felt bereft of choice, forced to live by rules I disagreed with—curfews, dress codes, chores. My sisters had helped me to perfect a range of infuriated sulks, pouts, and related bad moods, which I employed at the slightest affront, since arguing with Dad never made a dent in his demands. By seventh grade, I saw myself as Spokane's oldest altar boy with the shortest haircut—a sore thumb in a blousy cassock. I most resented my father while in church: me kneeling at Father Austen's feet, ready to ring the bell as he raised the chalice—"This is the body of Christ"—Dad watching overhead from the raised pulpit.

Buzzzzzzz.

I sprang from my knees like a sprinter off the blocks. Dad drove us to the plant and handed me over to Smitty, who paired me with a driver who showed me the ropes for several days—loading the truck, driving it, unloading product, filling orders at stores, stocking vending machines, picking up empties, doing paperwork. He showed me everything, yet never let me *do* much. I'm sure I would've just slowed him down. Anyway, I knew the real learning would come when I was on my own.

Indeed. There I am a week later, having successfully loaded my truck and left the plant, my day's route mapped out, waiting at a red light a block away on Monroe, a slightly inclining street, headed north. I was rather proud of myself. The light turned green. I eased up on the clutch and down on the gas and the world gently floated backward. I slammed on the brake before hitting the car behind me and lost contact with the clutch. The truck sputtered, snorted, then died. I pulled the emergency brake and started it up again. As before, when I tried to ease into first gear, the truck rolled back. In the side mirror, I saw cars behind me streaming into the other lane, all honking. I felt like a circus midget atop a lumbering old elephant, the crowd roaring at my ineptitude. The light turned red, I took a deep breath, and prepared to start over. The truck lurched back. This continued six or eight times, until I found I'd rolled all the way down the hill. I was positioned on Monroe directly in front of the Coke plant. I considered abandoning the truck right there, going into the plant, and getting Smitty to help me. But I was back on flat ground, and in a final attempt, I got into first gear. I sailed through a yellow light and on into town.

I probably had more fender benders in my truck over those three summer months than my one-eyed father has ever had in a car. The freeway was fine; it was grocery-store parking lots that were the most hazardous for me. By midsummer, I'd earned a nickname from the other drivers: Crash. And when I left the job to start my senior year of high school, they gave me a helmet as a present. I considered it a trophy. By all rights, I should have been fired right off, but I did manage always to get the Coke delivered and the empty bottles picked up. That's what mattered. I was relieved not to work there any longer, yet there were things about the job I loved, not the least of which was the money. Also, my route changed all the time, as I took over when men went on vacation, so I got to drive all over the Inland Empire. Often I was assigned "scrap runs"—small deliveries that took so much time, no one else wanted to do them. I thought these were the most fun. At the end of a long drive into rural northern Idaho, for instance, I tracked down a tiny mom-and-pop grocery, where they gave me free pie and ice cream. My trip to an Indian reservation near Walla Walla was met by a gaggle of screaming kids delighted to see the Coke man.

I was happy being by myself, driving, with the radio cranked up, the windows rolled down. If I finished deliveries early, I'd stop at Lake Coeur d'Alene, smoke a joint, and go swimming in my underwear. I'd be back at the plant by 4 P.M. to clock out. As a sophomore, I'd begun buying homegrown pot from the older brother of a classmate. I hid it under a removable bottom shelf in my bathroom cabinet together with a bong, pipe, and rolling papers. I treasured all the paraphernalia of drug use, the myriad accessories for secretly being bad.

While I rebelled by getting stoned, I also tried to fit in by having a girlfriend. On weekends, Teri and I would sometimes get high and have sex in the attic of her house. Though we'd share a bed, I could never go so far as to fall asleep. I was amazed that she could doze off beside me; I couldn't sustain that level of intimacy. I lived with a fear of getting caught—not caught in bed with Teri (that didn't concern me much at all) but in a lie about myself. Never far from every waking thought was the desire for men.

Back home by my 1 A.M. curfew, I'd sometimes remain awake the rest of the night, holed up in my room, listening to records at a whisper's decibel. My father was often awake those nights, too. This fact seems kind of sad now, and emblematic of our relationship: we were two insomniacs under the same roof, yet we never kept each other company.

Of course, this is a sentimental notion, completely at odds with the reality of being a teenager and, for that matter, of being the father of a teenage son. I didn't want anything to do with him at that age. And he didn't know what to make of me. On sleepless nights, I would never have gone upstairs, except to steal Scotch from his liquor cabinet. (I recall making a ghastly concoction of warm milk and Johnnie Walker.) If he had come down to my room—a candlelit shrine to female singer-songwriters and male bodybuilders—I would have gotten rid of him as quickly as possible.

In fairness, I should also add that my father hotly denies he's ever had much trouble sleeping. ("What is it you call me?" he said, grinning, during a recent visit. "An unsomniac? Kleptomaniac? Some damn thing!" I laughed and teased him, "Yeah, that's close: you're an unseemly kleptomaniac.") He thinks I'm nuts. But my story stands. One thing insomnia has given me is good hearing in the dark. I remember the sound of his footsteps overhead as clearly as his comments the next morning ("Didn't sleep worth a damn").

The Coca-Cola plant, like caffeinated Coke syrup itself, must have provided the raw material for years of sleepless nights. Working for him in the summer of 1978 left me with this unforgettable impression. Although we had little contact after the morning's drive to work, I caught occasional glimpses of him *at* work, leading meetings, zipping around the plant, making sales calls. He worked hard. He'd worked hard for a long time. And it was becoming difficult to survive financially. In a small, competitive market, where canned beverages and plastic containers were more popular, far cheaper, and much easier to transport and store than bottles, glass was becoming a thing of the past. Early the next summer, fifteen years after we'd moved from Minneapolis, Dad had to sell the pop factory. His dream that someday I'd work full-time for the family business, as he once had for his father, quietly died.

Any hope he had that I'd follow in his footsteps as a West Point cadet had fizzled many years earlier. Following my high school graduation, the only serious pressure I felt from Dad was to study business at college rather than poetry. I had chosen Santa Clara University, about an hour south of San Francisco, primarily because it was located in California. My father was satisfied that it met his main requirement: it was a Catholic school. Entrusted to the Jesuits, I left for college in September of 1979 and, at age fifty-five, he moved on to another job.

≈

Jet Lag

J ET LAG is justice. Insomniacs such as myself secretly enjoy nothing more than the temporary suffering of our loved ones who sleep perfectly at home. It affects even the most gifted specimens—those who treat sleep as recreation, something they can choose to do whenever and wherever they so desire, and have no shame about demonstrating this freakish ability on buses, beaches, and in other public places. If they cross at least three time zones by plane, they will end up with a touch of jet lag. It's the turista of good sleepers. Accompany them to Europe or, better yet, on a spiritual journey from North America to India: after an eighteen-hour flight, they, too, will learn what it is like to have sleepless nights and to be swamped by fatigue in the middle of the day. They will feel the jelly legs, achy joints, and generalized malaise of a chronic insomniac, as if drunk on their own body chemistry. There's not a prayer in the world that can help them. They may find themselves half-mad at 3 A.M., begging for a sedative. To which the insomniac can say, "How 'bout a nice, plump, pink-and-red Restoril? Here, take two. Wash 'em down with a swig of warm beer. Nighty-night. Can't wait to see you in the morning."

It is sweet revenge for all their patronizing past comments—words that the insomniac can wickedly throw back at them: *Gosh, you look so tired. You've got to relax. Have you tried chamomile tea? A hot bath? Aromatherapy? Don't think about it so much. Gee, I slept fine. Maybe you're overreacting. . . .* Sweet, yet short-lived. Good sleepers who are also sensible and patient, as they all seem to be, will adjust to jet lag. They'll be taking siesta with the locals—napping on park benches, for God's sake—all too soon.

It's not all fun and games for insomniacs, of course. Jet lag is another few nights of the same poison, just at a stronger dose. In some ways, I think we do handle it better than good sleepers, during daytime at least, because we're more used to being sleep-deprived. Not that we enjoy it. Jet lag can bring out the worst in us—well, not jet lag per se, but traveling: all of our sleep phobias and obsessive-compulsive routines rush to the surface as predictably as a tourist's sunburn on the first day at the beach. Sleep is difficult enough in one's own home. To adjust to an unfamiliar bedroom, mattress, headboard, sheets, blankets, pillows (and this is assuming one has a proper bed, not a couch or rollaway, to sleep on)—it can be more unnerving than driving on the autobahn in a rental car and trying to read the signs in German. There are so many things to consider at bedtime—is the darkness sufficient, room temperature perfect, weather conducive, silence pervasive, or noise negligible enough? Is the mattress just so? Bedspread on or off? Window open or closed? All conditions have to be right. A jet-lagged insomniac could count backward the number of obstacles to falling asleep and never get drowsy.

Jet lag—rather unique among the insomnias, parasomnias, and hypersomnias comprised in the world of sleep medicine—is a recent phenomenon, far more so than "shift-work sleep disorder," a related syndrome, whose roots can be traced to the industrial revolution, when refineries and foundries began to stay open around the clock. Jet lag arrived with the jet age of the 1950s (made possible by the development of the jet engine during World War II), when commercial air travel started edging out trains or steamers as the quickest, most convenient and comfortable means for crossing a country or ocean. It was not named, and thereby broadly recognized as a legitimate physiological condition, until around 1969. Until then, jet lag was thought to be psychosomatic in nature, a common complaint, like "flight nerves." Dr. Kleitman, in the 1963 edition of *Sleep and Wakefulness,* never addressed it.

Now jet lag is understood universally and studied seriously, and it goes by a variety of titles: circadian desynchronosis or transmeridian flight desynchronosis or time zone change syndrome. They all mean one thing: the body's internal clock is out of sync with the external time cues, or zeitgebers, that normally guide it, such as sunlight and darkness. What we think of as one clock is actually an interconnected complex of hundreds, perhaps thousands, of different clocks, or cycles, which run in all cells, tissues, and organs of the human body, each with its own function and frequency. Circadian cycles, such as sleep and wakefulness, are daily, while "ultradian" cycles are much shorter, ranging from the release of hormones, which may last several hours, to the electrical activity of the brain, which runs in fractions of a second. "Infradian" cycles are longer than twenty-four hours, such as the approximately monthly cycle of menstruation. There are cycles within cycles, too. Each individual sleep stage, for example, is a discrete ultradian cycle.

The existence of a biological clock in nature was proved in 1955 by the eminent Austrian zoologist Karl von Frisch, an expert in bees. In work begun thirty years earlier, he found that he could train bees to feed at a specific time during the day. Dr. von Frisch was surprised both by how easy this conditioning was and by the insects' punctuality. He assumed they possessed an internal "time sense." To eliminate the chance that the bees were somehow using the sun as a timepiece, he repeated the training in an underground mine. Again, he was successful, though he thought they could also be detecting a form of solar radiation unknown to humans. To test this further, he trained a group of bees in Germany, then shipped them across the Atlantic with one of his assistants. Would they keep feeding at German time or adapt to local time as the boat traveled west? Dr. von Frisch's young assistant became so seasick during the voyage that she could not carry out the experiment. Then World War II erupted and his research was suspended for many years.

It may have been for the best, as Dr. von Frisch recalled in his memoir; the great advancements in air travel after the war allowed him to improve the experiment. In 1955, he tried again. Because the best flight connections to New York were from Paris, he asked a French colleague to train a hive of bees. Conditioned to a certain feeding time in a dark room in Paris, they were then packed into a dark box and flown across the Atlantic. After they arrived in the United States, another colleague expedited their clearance through customs and took them straight to a dark room at the American Museum of Natural History. "Twenty-four hours after their last meal in Paris," the doctor wrote, "they punctually turned up at their little food dish in New York. This proved without a doubt that they possessed an internal clock."

That humans have a comparable timekeeping mechanism was not recognized until the mid-1960s, and it wasn't until the early seventies that scientists began to focus on the phenomenon of jet lag. Many studies were supported by NATO, NASA, the air force, and the FAA, whose pilots and personnel were dangerously affected by this malady. They found that several conditions contribute to its severity. Jet lag is worse when flying east than west; it does not result from flights north or south. By losing eight hours, say, on an eastward flight, one's normal day is compacted and it's far more difficult to jump ahead to alter the sleep-wake cycle. For this same reason, daylight saving time during the spring, when an hour is lost, presents a more difficult adjustment than the return to standard time in the fall. (In a sense, the internal clock "expands" better than it "contracts.") Adjusting to jet lag requires one day for every time zone crossed.

It's common for people to sleep poorly the night before traveling; this pretrip insomnia may exacerbate the effects of jet lag. Conditions on the plane also rarely help, such as the stress and discomfort caused by long, crowded flights. Nodding off in your seat only adds to the problem, in my opinion. Sleeping in your clothes, upright, squeezed- and strapped-in, somehow makes you more tired; it's no better than snoozing on a hard, dirty floor. Fear of flying can exact a terrible price, too, as can claustrophobia or acrophobia; shattered nerves do not heal upon landing. Reduced oxygen and low humidity in the cabin—on top of consuming alcohol, sleeping pills, or caffeine—may also explain why some passengers feel doubly sick and tired as they stumble off a plane.

All kinds of remedies have been suggested for alleviating jet lag, including a jet lag diet or taking melatonin tablets before and after travel according to a precise schedule. Experts say that the most effective method is to actively set, or "entrain," your circadian clock to local zeitgebers once you reach your destination. There are "social zeitgebers" such as mealtimes, but daylight is the most potent influence. Nearly all of the body's cycles are set by the brain's suprachiasmatic nucleus (SCN), which is guided by geophysical correlates such as the earth's rotation, and the rising and setting sun. The SCN's function was verified in 1972 by two independent groups of scientists who used radiographic tracers to follow the path of light from the eyes to the hypothalamus, where the SCN is located. More recently, neuroscientists have proved that the SCN will still keep time even after it's taken out of a lab animal's brain or when transplanted from one into another.

I find that astounding: the essential mechanism for the body's clock is a discrete thing, pulsing with energy, something that can be removed and, theoretically, replaced, like a quartz battery. I would love to see the SCN floating in its warm petri dish: a tiny cluster of nerve cells, shaped like a boomerang, I'm told, as prosaic in a way as the coiled spring of an ordinary watch. The SCN is just one of many pieces, yet without it none of the others work. It is the key to a human's sense of time, of a day's passing. Which is to say, of one's sense of being alive.

My first bad case of jet lag came with my first trip abroad, of which my earliest clear impression still has the force and mass of something felt physically. Ten days into the trip, I'd shrugged off the last tendrils of jet lag from the nine time zones I'd crossed. It was a warm September evening in 1981. Shortly before, I had arrived by bus with ninety other students in Florence, Italy, where I was to spend my junior year of college. I'd left my luggage at the pensione where I would be living, smoked a joint, and gone for a walk, blindly making my way through the city's narrow alleys and streets as night fell. I couldn't see beyond the street I was walking on, nor much overhead. One street led into another, and another, until all at once it was as if a curtain parted; I stood at the edge of a large, brightly lit square, swarming with people. Before me, all of life seemed to be revolving around one massive stone building, the city's great domed cathedral, Il Duomo, faced in delicate green and white marble. I had practically smacked right into it. It was like going down a zigzagging cobblestone chute and landing not simply in a different time zone but headfirst in another time: the fifteenth century.

I felt ecstatically disoriented, a sensation that lasted all year. The cathedral, with its terra-cotta-tiled roof and tall, narrow bell tower, became the compass point for finding my way wherever I wanted to go, night or day. *Dovè il Duomo?* was one of the few complete sentences I knew how to say. I arrived knowing hardly any Italian, having failed my last semester of Italian at Santa Clara University. I hid the truth about my grades, lest my parents decide I shouldn't be allowed to go.

In fact, it had been their idea. My mother had toured Europe with some girlfriends after college in the fifties; three of my older sisters had spent their junior year in Florence; and my parents had visited several times. They were extraordinarily generous in making it possible for me. I chipped in my savings from school and summer jobs, but I was there on their dime, as I had been at Santa Clara. While studying Italian, Renaissance art, Shakespeare, and other liberal arts courses at school—housed in a palazzo not far from the Ponte Vecchio—I traveled on weekends and breaks with a Eurail pass. Over the year, I saw much of Italy and France and scattered cities in other countries—Germany, Austria, Israel, Greece, Egypt, Ireland, and the Soviet Union.

Little of my actual travels made it into the journal I kept all year. Characteristically, I was more interested in observing how I *felt* than what I saw; in recording how I slept than what I did during the day. I also enjoyed listing the most uncomfortable places I'd made a bed for myself: under a bench in the

Milan train station, for instance, or on a packed overnight train from Cairo to Luxor on my birthday. What started as a bout of jet lag, after flying from Spokane to Calgary to Frankfurt, turned into an ongoing struggle to get a single good night's sleep. This problem was doubtless compounded by the fact that I shared a small room in Florence with two other guys. Upon our arrival, the school administrators held a lottery for rooms and roommates. We'd all come from different schools and few of us previously knew one another. I ended up with a low number and no choice whatsoever. As the pool narrowed I remember thinking, *I could live with anyone here, anyone, except for Ben or Todd,* who had become friends on the weeklong bus trip from Frankfurt to Florence and distinguished themselves as the loudest, most obnoxious and most frequently drunk in a particularly loud and obnoxious group of drunk young Americans. I suspect they picked me as their roommate for the very reason I thought they never would: I was a quiet, well-mannered loner. It would be two against one.

I was also good cover for Ben and Todd, though I certainly wasn't above getting drunk and into trouble. I just didn't get caught—or arrested, as each of them did once. Assigned to the pensione farthest from school, we shared close, noisy quarters, an experience that disabused me of a lifelong fantasy of having brothers. Ben played the older one: the son of an American diplomat, raised in London, he had a British accent and more experience and money than any of the rest of us. Tall and lanky, he always wore Frye boots and a trench coat; sometimes he woke up in bed still wearing them. At a bar near school, the Coinca Café, he would drink negroni's, smoke Marlboros, and tell stories about wild summer vacations on the island of Elba or ski trips in Switzerland with his jet-set girlfriends. He was smooth and slippery. At twenty-one, Ben had the bulging eyes, sallow skin, and the purply, puckered lips of a poisoned codfish. He probably already had liver disease, he drank so much.

Todd played the younger brother: a small, scrappy punk with a mouth suited for a much larger head, his primary purpose for coming to Europe was to follow the Grateful Dead. He was always broke. Todd and his girlfriend, Maureen, joined other Deadheads on drug runs to Amsterdam and then disappeared for days at a time, returning with loopy stories about the latest concert. "It was fucking incredible," he'd say, lighting up a spliff near the window. "You should've been there." By which he did not mean a city visited, but an acid trip taken.

Todd's corner of the room was plastered with Grateful Dead posters. Ben's walls were empty; he couldn't be bothered. Mine held a map and a display of posters from the Uffizi, the Jeu d'Paume, and the Pompidou Center. I was the withdrawn, artistic middle brother, who was often spacing out in the corner, writing in a journal. I grew a beard and assumed the uniform of a student traveler: boots, army pants, flannel shirt. I spent much of my time plugged into "head tunes," a Walkman, which I considered the greatest technological advancement of the twentieth century; it transformed a body I loathed and mistrusted into something both beautiful and functional: a mobile stereo console. Music pouring into my ears, Joni Mitchell, Rickie Lee Jones, Patti Smith, X, and The Pretenders traveled inside of me.

Raised with five sisters, I was more comfortable around girls. Not long into the school year, I fell in love with one: a free-spirited blonde from Houston. The first time we had sex was on a weekend in Saint Francis's birthplace, Assisi. Our affair lasted precisely four weeks. It ended when she simultaneously realized she might be pregnant by her previous boyfriend and started an affair with a new one, my roommate Ben. I walked in on them. I was crushed and humiliated, yet buoyed by the growing evidence that I might, in fact, be straight, that my deviant past was just a bad memory. This tantalizing possibility preoccupied me for the rest of the year.

Insomnia struck differently then than it does now. Exhausted and often intoxicated, I could fall asleep right away, but I usually woke in the middle of the night. That's when I got to know Florence. My bed was right next to the door; at 4 A.M., I would pull on warm clothes and slip out with my backpack, Walkman, and passport (in case I decided to hop on a train). With my head tunes on, I existed in my own world. I felt safe and powerful, fluent in the vernacular of a sleeping city.

I walked from our pensione down to the open market, where vendors were setting up for the day. The square was lit by strings of bare bulbs. Tucked into a shadow, I'd sit on a curb and watch. It was like being on the grounds of a weird underworld circus in which all the animals were carcasses. The butchers were beautiful men, placing a kiss on each other's cheek as they said good morning. Families set up stands for fruit, root vegetables, flowers. Cafés opened before dawn, and I'd stop for a cappuccino and a sugary roll, savoring the warmth and the friendliness of the people gathered there. I didn't care that I didn't know the language well. I liked being outside the conversation, an eavesdropper with an excuse not to talk. Heading back out, I'd walk to the Duomo, then through Piazza Signoria, under the gaze of Hercules and Neptune and Perseus. After crossing the Ponte Vecchio, I'd climb the hill to Piazzale Michelangelo, where I could watch the sun come up.

I didn't walk to exhaust myself, but to be at my most lucid. Wandering around Florence helped to satisfy a craving for solitude. I was driven by it, yet could rarely find it in the way I pictured. It was akin to being cold to the bone and unable to get warm enough. An empty park at 6 A.M. overlooking the Arno River was a good place to disappear to, as was a train compartment full of strangers. In February, when there were fewer tourists, I discovered I could find it in a museum: the Accademia, which housed Michelangelo's *David*.

In small pockets of time in between crowds, I could be alone in the sunlit rotunda. I circled the room, like the second hand on a clock, studying him. An object of desire when I was thirteen, he had a different, deeper effect on me at twenty-one. A beautiful boy made by a man, David embodied the ideal masculinity. He was a figure of courage and calm, so impossibly perfect, he could not ever have been a work-in-progress, only a finished form, as if Michelangelo had approached a block of marble, held out his hand, and David had simply stepped forth: "Where would you like me to stand?" In his presence, I thought I'd never felt so peaceful. But then a guard returned or tourists rushed in or I had to get to class. My minute was up and soon the year would be, too. I'd have to go back home. I wished to return as someone new.

I felt much less like David than like one of Michelangelo's unfinished "captives" in the next gallery, twisting in stone. A crude chipping-away of my self had begun eighteen months earlier as I'd started my sophomore year at Santa Clara. I'd gotten involved with a man named Malcolm, an attorney who lived near campus. It occurs to me now that he bore a resemblance to my Florence roommate Ben—tall and leathery, with bloodshot eyes and blow-dried hair. More distinctive than his appearance was Malcolm's bed, a king-size fourposter. It looked like an overturned dining room table, one that had accommodated many guests. I don't think I even knew Malcolm's last name. All I had to do was ring his doorbell at any time of the night; he took care of the rest. Poppers and cocaine were included with the price of admission. I was so disassociated from my body, and so high, I could have claimed I was never there. The only decision I had to make was when to leave, which was between one and ten minutes after orgasm.

Later in the year, I met another man, Ron, also a graduate of Santa Clara's law school. It wasn't that I was attracted to older gay men; I never met or knew of any my own age. I didn't think many existed. Ron pursued me like a boyfriend. He called me at the dorm and took me on dates. Past thirty, he had a wounded, dejected air; I was, I admit, exactly the type to keep him that way. I lied and was cruel to him. If I saw him at the campus gym where we'd met, I wouldn't say hello. I stood him up or canceled plans at the last minute. When I didn't, I insisted that we meet off-campus and go places far from Santa Clara. For a while, a Mexican restaurant off the freeway near Mountain View, where they wouldn't card me, became the site for an occasional dinner. We sat in a booth in the back. I'd order the same thing every time—a beef tostada, served in an extravagant bowl-shaped shell, as big as a helmet. I was so nervous that someone I knew might walk in, I could never eat it. I filled up on giant frozen margaritas.

I wasn't completely paranoid. A rumor that I was gay had started making its way around the school. A girl asked me about it directly while I was standing in line in the meal hall; indignant, I denied it. The question came up again at a couple of parties. I had a few wonderful stoner friends who might have understood, but I was wary of the football-team jocks with whom we shared a dorm. One night I found "fag" scrawled on my door. I locked myself inside and lay awake until morning listening for taunts in the hall. I seriously considered killing myself. I could get pills to do it.

I was sufficiently enamored of Sylvia Plath, Anne Sexton, and other self-destructive artists to view suicide as a romantic end, but I also thought it would be an admission of guilt. Nothing could have pried me from my secret. I clung to it, in part, because I didn't really know myself what it meant to be a "fag." It was as if I had the address for a place, yet no map. Ron tried to show me how to get there. In a way that I didn't understand at the time—indeed, that I resisted—he introduced me to gay culture, the gay community. Although he didn't live in San Francisco, he wore the uniform of a "Castro

clone": button-fly Levi's, Izod shirt, clipped mustache, a diamond post in one ear. He talked to me about "coming out." He
told me about "the baths." He took me to a gay bar: the Boot
Rack Saloon. For years after, I saved an empty matchbook—
"Where San Jose's Men Go," it promised in silver ink on a
glossy black cover—but I've forgotten exactly where it was and
I wouldn't know where to begin looking now. What I do remember is walking through the door.

It was a sunny weekday afternoon, but inside the dark,
windowless bar it was night. The floor was cement and the
walls were painted orange. Colored paper lanterns hung from
corner to corner of the small, enclosed patio at the back. To
get my bearings, I headed toward something familiar: a drink.
My eyes adjusted to the murky candlelight.

The bartender wore a torn white tank top and tight white
jeans; a red bandanna was stuffed in his back pocket. I saw my
face in the mirrored wall behind the bar; above it were posters
of naked men with enormous erections. Next to the beer
glasses, a big can of Crisco was displayed aside a vase of flowers and a dildo studded with silver prongs. I glimpsed a man in
a leather jacket leaning against the back patio wall, holding
someone's head against his legs. Someone else was waiting his
turn. I turned around on the barstool toward Ron, who put his
arm around my shoulder. So this is what it's like, I thought, at
once resigned and relieved: I was not afraid to kiss him here.

I was drunk when we got back to his apartment. He gave
me a towel and told me to go to the bathroom to wash up. I
didn't know what I was supposed to do with it. I was scared
and excited: this was my final initiation, as much a symbolic
act as a sexual one, and I just wanted to do it, to get fucked,
something I'd avoided until then. When I returned to the bedroom, he was sitting on the bed with his clothes off. "Do you
want me to turn out the light?" was my only question. Asking
him to use a condom never occurred to me.

Ron leaned over me to take a bottle of lotion from the bedside table. "Here," he said, vigorously shaking the bottle, and poured a puddle of cold, pale yellow cream into the palm of my hand. He shook the bottle over his crotch and pulled his penis up into the air, stretching it like a piece of sticky, glistening taffy, dropping and stretching it up again, until it became hard. Then he reached for the light.

A week later, we were to have another date, yet for the first time I wasn't the one who canceled. Ron did. He called to say he was sick—chills and a fever, 105 degrees. Within a few days, I also got a call from Malcolm, whom I had not seen in months. He thought he might have hepatitis or something—he, too, had terrible flu symptoms. At his suggestion, I went to a clinic but I checked out fine. My sophomore year ended a couple weeks later and I never saw Ron or Malcolm again. In June of 1981, I drove to Spokane for the summer before going to Europe.

I was twenty years old when I arrived in Florence, the same age as Nathaniel Kleitman when he'd come to the United States. Few further similarities exist between us. He had been a Zionist immigrant and a medical student in Palestine. Photographs show he had a full, round face, thick, dark hair, a husky build. During World War I, when the ruling Turks forced Russians out of the country, he and other refugees had taken flight and were picked up in Rhodes by a battleship, *The Des Moines*. With such a name, he first thought the ship had to be headed for a French port. Instead, in 1915, Nathaniel Kleitman had arrived at Ellis Island. He hardly knew a soul in the United States and spoke virtually no English. He had no particular intention of staying, Dr. Kleitman has said in an interview; he just needed a safe place to live while the war was going on. In this, I notice a parallel in our journeys: each changed the course of a young man's life and quite possibly saved it.

Chapter 12

✢

Asleep Awake

I SAW MY stay in Europe as a reprieve, a yearlong break from my battles with myself, a conception modeled closely, I should add, after the lyrical theme of Joni Mitchell's album *Hejira*—a flight from love's dangers. In my mind, I was able to escape the life I'd led and dream up a new, rootless one, in which I abstained from homosexuality. In fact, the reprieve was real, though in a way I could never have known or imagined. On June 5, 1981, just days after I had last heard from Ron, the Centers for Disease Control had published what would later be recognized as the first report on the AIDS epidemic: five puzzling cases in Los Angeles of *Pneumocystis carinii* pneumonia in homosexual men. Similar cases then surfaced in New York and San Francisco. By the summer of

1982, when I returned to the States, the disease was named; the small outbreak had grown to nearly five hundred cases nationally; and at least a hundred gay men were dead, with thousands more infected, Ron and Malcolm among them, I felt certain. I could have been, too, had I not spent the year in Florence.

Returning to Santa Clara University for my senior year, I didn't fall back into my circle of friends in the same way. I moved into an apartment and resumed my studies as an English major, focusing seriously for the first time on poetry and fiction writing. While desiring men no less, I didn't act on it and was no longer dogged by rumors of being gay. At the start of the school year, I found a new girlfriend, a young, militant Muslim Palestinian and aspiring actress from Jordan. Oh, my. We didn't really have much in common, except a love of dramatic theater.

Although I completed a manuscript of poetry that won a statewide competition, senior year was a bit late to turn my academic life around. I wanted to go on to graduate school in creative writing, yet knew I wouldn't get a scholarship—I had raised my grades, but they were just average. My parents were not inclined to continue supporting me financially, nor was I inclined to ask for their support, a principle that became an imperative when my father suddenly lost his management job a couple weeks before I was to graduate. In the spring of 1983, I found myself facing an economic crisis as much as an identity crisis, hardly unique for someone my age and with all the advantages I'd enjoyed: What was I going to do with my life?

Employment prospects for myself were grim; it was the Reagan era, the country was heading into a recession, and the trend was to avoid the job market and get an MBA, which did not interest me. I'd been working part-time for a courier service, using my Volkswagen to make deliveries in Silicon Valley, but I only scraped by. A series of interviews with IBM for a job writing computer manuals left me resolute that I would not take any work that might bruise my creativity. And although I'd had a senior-year internship at a news-radio station in San Francisco, I never went after a permanent position; the office was on Polk Street, in a gay neighborhood, and the temptations it presented were too great.

I affected an image of myself styled after the heroines of Joan Didion novels (never mind that I was male): a heavily sedated character for whom extreme passivity served as a survival strategy. Like Grace Strasser-Mendana in my favorite work, *A Book of Common Prayer,* I was aloof, watchful, and imperturbable, "a student of delusion," yet not wise or ironic enough to see that it was myself by which I was deluded. Incapable of making up my mind, I let my parents decide for me: I would move back home for the summer to save on expenses. It's the right thing to do, I told myself. I broke up with my girlfriend of eight months and loaded up the car.

The only thing I was sure about when I arrived in Spokane was that I was very, very tired. Tired of saying good-byes to people, tired of being conflicted, tired of secrets, tired from driving. I moved my boxes into the dim, cool basement room I'd first lived in as a sixteen-year-old. How strange to be back inside that egg. I collapsed into bed, feeling fragile but safe.

I had always kept one small space within myself protected, shut off; that night, I could feel it opening up, like a dark sinkhole, swallowing me. When I woke up ten or twelve hours later, I was sick. I had swollen lymph nodes, a high fever, and was so exhausted that I could barely get out of bed. I was soon diagnosed by our family physician, Dr. Porter, with old-fashioned "kissing disease," mononucleosis. A common viral infection, mononucleosis is untreatable; bed rest is the only cure.

Sleep was irresistible; neither enjoyable nor refreshing, but effortless in a way that I'd never before known. I nodded off while talking, while sitting up in bed. I fell in and out of feverish sleep, never paying attention to day or night. It overtook every desire: hunger, thirst, sex. And every fear. I couldn't think about anything. Buried under sheets, blankets, comforter, it was as if time had stopped, my life had stopped, and I could rest.

While I did not consciously will myself to become sick, I welcomed the delirious, all-consuming drowsiness. I was helpless to it, science would explain. The body is rigged to sleep when it's ill or wounded: cytokines, acting as chemical messengers of the immune system, rally infection-fighting lymphocytes and induce slumber. The reverse also occurs: without adequate sleep, lymphocytes are reduced, thereby depressing the immune system. This explains why students often get sick during final exams, when they "pull all-nighters," or why a jag of insomnia ends with a nasty cold.

For some people, excessive sleep—which scientists call hypersomnia—is a response to stress or trauma, exactly like its antithesis, insomnia. Napoleon, who prided himself on only needing four hours of sleep per night, reputedly fell into a deep slumber after losing the battle of Aspern, his first defeat after seventeen victories. So overcome was he by this failure, he slept for thirty-six hours without awakening, according to the Russian scientist Marie de Manacéine.

Napoleon's was a rare case, de Manacéine hastened to add. Most instances of excessive sleep, she wrote in 1897, were the result of a "feebly developed consciousness," which could be found only in children, the lower classes, and in "savages, cretins, and people of inferior intelligence." She wasn't the first doctor to view hypersomnia as a sign of stupidity or insanity, nor the last, but may have been one of the cruelest. De Manacéine treated it with a form of electroshock therapy, something I daresay she enjoyed. Electricity acted, she reported, like a "gymnastics of the blood." I can practically smell the singed human hair, together with the scent of Madame de Manacéine's morning coffee and cigarette, as she jolts another patient awake in her St. Petersburg laboratory.

Robert MacNish, in practice in Glasgow some seventy years earlier, sounded like a much more sympathetic doctor. "There are persons who have a disposition to sleep on every occasion," he noted in a lively chapter on drowsiness in *The Philosophy of Sleep*. "They do so at all times and in all places. They sleep after dinner; they sleep in the theatre; they sleep in church. . . . Morpheus is the deity at whose shrine they worship—the only god whose influence over them is omnipotent." While Dr. MacNish did, on occasion, attempt to cure persistent drowsiness with laxatives and bloodletting, he felt that such cases were mainly without remedy, "for the soporific tendency springs from some natural defect, which no medicinal means can overcome." One particular phrase the doctor used to describe these patients sticks out: "It falls upon them in the midst of mirth." This observation is far less whimsical when one realizes that Dr. MacNish was likely describing narcoleptics, in whom attacks can be brought on by a fit of laughter.

Not formally identified until 1880 by the French physician Jean Baptiste Edouard Gélineau, who coined the term, narcolepsy is characterized by irresistible attacks of sleep. The episodes may last only thirty seconds or stretch to thirty minutes or more. Gélineau made his first diagnosis in a Parisian wine-barrel merchant, whom others had long thought was just a drunk, for he was a jolly man who loved to laugh; consequently, he often appeared to pass out in public. A precise understanding of narcolepsy only surfaced once brain waves could be measured and sleep stages differentiated. Narcolepsy is a disabling brain disorder marked by the sudden intrusion of REM sleep into wakefulness. The bouts of sleep, hundreds daily in some cases, are often triggered by excitement or emotional outbursts, which cause a sudden weakness or paralysis of the muscles—a condition called cataplexy.

Attacks may be subtle or extreme. The person sitting next to you at a staff meeting, for instance, appears to fall asleep; his jaw sags, his head leans forward, his arms drop to his side. In a moment, he's awake again, none the worse for wear. Or, a driver is cut off. She shouts an invective. Then, in an instant, she's out like a light behind the wheel, her body pressing the horn, her car veering into oncoming traffic.

While people with normal sleep patterns progress to REM after about ninety minutes, narcoleptics fall right into it, day or night, exactly like babies do at sleep onset. This sleep is also often accompanied by intense hypnagogic hallucinations, like those a healthy person might have while falling asleep. An incurable, lifelong condition, slightly more common in males than females, narcolepsy can be partially controlled by combining a stimulant such as Modafinil (for the sleepiness) with an antidepressant (for the cataplexy). It is not a rare illness, with an estimated three to four narcoleptics for every ten thousand people. Although scientists have confirmed a clear genetic component to narcolepsy, other factors may also be involved. The first episode may follow a psychologically traumatic event, such as the death of a loved one, or a serious brain injury. Symptoms usually first appear in adolescence but may be misdiagnosed for years. A teenager's daytime sleepiness may be considered normal behavior and therefore either punished or ignored.

Of course, excessive sleep *can* be a sign of teenage indolence—oversleeping as an excuse, say, for missing church. And there is such a thing as a "Long Sleeper," one of ninety possible diagnoses listed in the International Classification of Sleep Disorders. (Yes, there are "Short Sleepers," too.) Being a Long Sleeper isn't any more grave or complex than it sounds; you just sleep more than what's considered normal. Excessive sleep is perhaps most likely to be a symptom of clinical depression—a way to escape reality in dreaming. This is by no means a modern phenomenon. At an 1884 meeting of the New York Neurological Society, for instance, a thirty-two-year-old physician, identified only by his initials, "G. P. S.," spoke at length about his personal struggle with this condition, then called "morbid somnolence." It started in medical school, Dr. S. said, according to the meeting minutes for May 6 (published in the *Journal of Nervous and Mental Disease*).

"I do not think there was a single day when I did not at least once during the lectures either go soundly asleep or pass into a state of semi-unconsciousness, in which, although I heard what was going on, I did not understand it." He also found that he could not read his textbooks for more than half an hour without falling asleep. It seems plausible that he was just terribly sleep-deprived, as is the typical med student today, yet the fatigue persisted even after he started his practice, and it struck at the most inopportune moments.

"I have gone to sleep while making a vaginal examination in case of labor," Dr. S. said, an admission that strongly suggests he was not simply overworked. He would seem to fit my definition for a nervous nellie: someone so timid and excitable as to be frightened by signs of life itself. But instead of passing out, Dr. S. nodded off. Clearly, the doctor was ill-suited to his profession and, as further comments would suggest, to his own body. "I am troubled occasionally—perhaps three or four times a month, although a few years ago it was two or three times a week—with nocturnal emissions and weeping penis," he added, while neglecting to define the latter condition. "And always after these occurrences my symptoms are worse."

If it was customary for the society members to applaud after a speaker finished, Dr. S.'s closing words probably dampened their enthusiasm: "Although I am never 'sick' I never feel very well and frequently feel life a burden." With that, he left the podium. The New York Neurological Society promptly moved on to hear a case of "unilateral spasm of the tongue" and then adjourned, without offering Dr. S. any advice. If only he could have written himself a prescription for Prozac! Instead, I imagine, Dr. S. went home alone and crawled into bed.

He and his weeping penis would have been an ideal case for Sigmund Freud, himself a trained neurologist, who was just beginning to develop his theories. Freud came to define sleep as a quintessentially narcissistic state in which there is "an almost complete withdrawal from the surrounding world and the cessation of all interest in it." In a 1916 paper, "Metapsychological Supplement to the Theory of Dreams," he observed that "every night human beings lay aside the garments they pull over their skin, and even also other objects which they use to supplement their bodily organs . . . for instance, their spectacles, false hair or teeth, and so on. In addition to this, when they go to sleep they perform a perfectly analogous dismantling of their minds . . . thus both physically and mentally approaching remarkably close to the situation in which they began life." Naked, their nightly regression to an "intra-uterine existence" is fulfilled, Freud believed, in the warmth of a bed, the darkness of night, and in the sleeper's repose, frequently taken in the fetal position.

Malcolm M. Willey, an American disciple of Freud's, took a more utilitarian view of sleep. In a 1924 issue of the *Journal of Abnormal Psychology*, he cited the perfectly normal-seeming case of "Alfred S.," a prosperous banker who would get "dead sleepy" every evening as he and his wife talked. It required only a brief analysis, Willey noted, to bring out that, for

Alfred, sleep was an antidote to sheer boredom. "It is the escape of a successful young man with an adventurous past, who, unconsciously perhaps, feels fettered by the monotony of a conventional, settled, family existence."

I have no reason to doubt that Alfred was bored, nor do I have the credentials to challenge Dr. Willey's analysis. Yet I am compelled to suggest that there may also have been a physiological basis for his excessive sleepiness. Alfred S. could have had obstructive sleep apnea syndrome (OSAS), a respiratory disorder that causes people to stop breathing for short periods while sleeping—sometimes hundreds of times per night. (A single apneic episode is a minimum of ten seconds without breathing.) Though it can be hereditary—in cases of big tongues and narrow throats, that is—obesity is the greatest risk factor for OSAS, which is most prevalent today among middle-aged men who are overweight and smoke. When their muscles relax with sleep, the soft tissue in the throat collapses and shuts off airways; they wake partially, gasping for breath. The throat opens briefly, like a camera lens at a slow shutter speed, and again snaps closed. This disrupted sleep leaves them feeling exhausted during the day, though they'll often have no idea why, especially if they sleep alone. People rarely remember apneic episodes come morning, but if they sleep with someone, they're sure to hear about it. Monstrous snoring is typical. Headaches, erectile dysfunction, and hypertension are other symptoms of OSAS, though unremitting daytime fatigue is most common. It can endanger others, too. Falling asleep at the wheel, whether because of OSAS, narcolepsy, or plain exhaustion, causes at least one hundred thousand car accidents, seventy-six thousand injuries, and fifteen hundred fatalities annually in the United States, according to the National Highway Traffic Safety Administration.

Over the past thirty-five years, advances in understanding obstructive sleep apnea have coincided with a rise in obesity. Today it is the most common disorder seen in sleep clinics around the world, although its prevalence varies from country to country, depending on the health of the population. In the United States, where one in five adults is obese—more than 30 percent over his or her ideal body weight—OSAS accounts for about 80 percent of the patients at sleep clinics. The syndrome is now treatable through a variety of means, including surgical procedures to widen the trachea, remove the uvula, and reduce tongue size, or a ventilator mask that continually forces air into a sleeping person's lungs, yet OSAS may remain life-threatening.

One can literally choke to death in his sleep. This is not, however, what Dr. Willey had in mind when he wrote about another patient, "Theo L.," in a 1924 issue of *Psychoanalytic Review*. In this case, Willey made a more sensational diagnosis: excessive sleep served as a form of "temporary suicide." A twenty-four-year-old college student, Theo started feeling drowsy all the time in the spring of his senior year. "He lived for hours each day in a semi-hypnagogic state," Willey wrote; Theo took two-hour naps each afternoon and slept twelve or more hours per night. "The boy fully realized that he was losing his grip upon himself," so he consulted the psychoanalyst. Unrequited love was the source of Theo's disorder, the doctor determined; an infatuation with a certain girl conflicted with a terrible fear that she would reject him. "To escape this there was the unconscious induction of sleepiness; for in sleep Theo escaped from his tormenting thoughts."

The other possibility is that young Theo had mononucleosis, his torment notwithstanding. The two are not mutually exclusive, as I discovered in my own case. The illness, first accurately identified in 1920, is caused by the Epstein-Barr virus (EBV), one of the most common human viruses in the world. Thought to be present in approximately 95 percent of the adult U.S. population, EBV is usually transmitted through saliva. Among college students, mononucleosis accounts for more days missed from school than any other infectious disease, a recent report states. Symptoms of "mono" seldom last more than three or four months; there are rare cases, however, in which the infection evolves into an incurable chronic illness called idiopathic central nervous system (CNS) hypersomnia.

CNS hypersomnia causes an unslakable daytime sleepiness, without the abrupt sleep attacks and cataplexy seen in narcolepsy. The disorder, identified only within the past twenty-five years, is further differentiated from narcolepsy by what seems to be a progressive eroding of neurologic functioning, a symptom that can be mistaken for mental illness. It may be a variant of a separate sleep disorder, the name of which sounds like an intriguing sci-fi book title, "the subwakefulness syndrome"; scientists have not come to a consensus on this point. According to Christian Guilleminault, a Stanford scientist who has done extensive research on these disorders, people with CNS hypersomnia begin to act like horror-film zombies. At once asleep and awake, with eyes open but blank, they may utter loud bursts of nonsensical speech, as if sleeptalking, or do inappropriate things without later remembering, such as traveling miles from home for no reason.

This strange, mindless behavior sets it apart from another enigmatic illness, chronic fatigue syndrome (CFS). People diagnosed with CFS often describe its onset as sudden but not alarming because many of its symptoms mimic those of the flu. And, in fact, it may start with the flu, a bad cold, or another viral infection. While such illnesses usually clear up after a few weeks, CFS persists for six months or more, perhaps never lifting. One's life becomes overwhelmed by a strain of tiredness that demands sleep, yet is not alleviated by it.

Contrary to a popular conception, CFS is not a new "yuppie flu." Similar if not identical syndromes, known by different names, date back at least 140 years. In the 1860s, Dr. George Beard labeled it neurasthenia, believing it to be a neurosis characterized by physical and mental fragility. A century later, it was called nervous exhaustion, a glamorous-sounding condition that seemed only to befall opera divas and movie stars; ordinary housewives just got "iron-poor blood." Such illnesses were always diagnosed far more frequently in women than in men, as is CFS today, the reasons for which may be physiological as well as cultural. A real gender difference could exist with CFS, similar to a disease such as lupus. At the same time, women may be more willing than men to consult doctors about symptoms of fatigue and weakness, and doctors may be more likely to diagnose women with "emotional problems." The root cause of CFS remains unknown, and the illness is without successful treatments, yet some people find relief of symptoms in antidepressant and antianxiety drugs. Which does not necessarily resolve anything. The question remains: Do shattered nerves lead in some cases to illness, or does illness lead to nervous exhaustion?

Right at the moment I should have been preparing to go out into the world, to become independent, at age twenty-two, I fell back into my parents' care. Before mono, I had never been that ill, nor even had stitches, for that matter. At home during the day, my father was constantly checking in on me, with the tenderness that only emerged when one of his kids got sick. For the first three weeks, I felt like a five-year-old again: Dad feeling my forehead for a temperature, Mom bringing me aspirin and a glass of Coca-Cola.

In one concentrated dose, they were providing everything I was about to lose, and not simply because I was now a grown man. One day soon, I realized in a single piercing thought while lying in bed, I had to tell them something that would devastate them and completely alter our relationship. The question was no longer *if* I should but *when* I would. I knew it wouldn't be that summer—that was too close, too soon. But, like a fever spiking, there was no stopping it. Having this knowledge in advance made their unconditional love and support, at present, almost unbearably painful.

All my defenses were down. My brain, usually wired against missteps like an alarm system, seemed on the fritz. I couldn't muster the strength to keep emotion at bay, nor make clear distinctions between what I knew to be true and what I'd dreamed in a fever. One day, Mom was in the room to make my bed; I slumped in a chair nearby. I took a deep breath, and when it came out, I completely broke down. I can see myself hunched over and hear myself wailing. How strange to be crying on a warm June afternoon, but I couldn't stop. For what felt like hours, but was probably thirty minutes, I was inconsolable.

What had set it off? Was it the loving gesture of my mother putting fresh sheets on my bed? I can still smell them as she snapped open the white sheets in the stale basement air, like an ampoule of oxygen broken under my nose. I can see her leaning over the mattress: she gently wrestled each corner into the taut fitted sheet, as though helping a child into his shirtsleeves.

She would have done anything to help me feel better, to shore me up. She always had. When I was growing up, she encouraged my writing and also shared her creativity with me—showing me how to paint and sculpt and how to film and edit silly 8mm movies. In late-night games of cribbage, just the two of us, when I might talk about books I was reading, and at local symphony concerts and plays, when I sometimes took Dad's place if he couldn't go, she made space for me to enjoy myself, to enjoy *being* myself, a feeling that now seemed impossibly far away. From deep inside, I was overwhelmed by shame. She held and quieted me, then put me to bed, tucking the top sheet in tight around my body like clean bandages.

I would have lain there forever if I could. Not moving, barely breathing. In sleep, I was still her boy, unchanged, like Endymion of Greek mythology, a young shepherd who fell asleep on Mount Latmus with the moon goddess, Selene, at his side. When he woke at daylight to find her gone, Endymion begged Zeus to grant him eternal sleep, for Selene had filled his head with the most wonderful dreams. Zeus obliged, and the boy's youth and beauty were forever preserved for the adoring moon.

Fond as I am of mythologizing, I cannot alter the facts of my story. After three weeks' rest, I was sick of sleep, glad to be getting out of bed. Nevertheless, it still took five more weeks to regain full health. As a broken bone is said to be stronger once mended, so too was my sense of myself. It was as though the bandages holding me together had loosened with wear; I could peek through the eye holes and feel my limbs stir.

In *The Philosophy of Sleep*, Dr. MacNish describes a case that would seem to me far-fetched if it did not in a certain way resemble my own. "The subject was a young lady, of a good constitution, excellent capacity, and well educated," he wrote. "Her memory was capacious and well stored with a copious stock of ideas. Unexpectedly, and without any forewarning, she fell into a profound sleep. On waking, she was discovered to have lost every trait of acquired knowledge. Her memory was *tabula rasa*—all vestiges, both of words and things, were obliterated and gone. It was found necessary for her to learn everything again." Her transformation was a mystery to her family, yet to her it was quite plain, Dr. MacNish noted. "The former condition of her existence she now calls the Old State," while every event and occurrence since then was "New."

By late August, I knew exactly what I was going to do. Before talking with my parents, I would become financially independent and begin living as an out gay man. I made plans to move to Seattle, where three of my sisters were living, and to find a job. My parents were making changes of their own. With my younger sister in college, they had just put the family home up for sale. I packed my bed and other furniture into a U-Haul trailer and moved out. As I left Spokane, I felt the bandage layers begin to unravel, trailing like a long, long white scarf out the car window, over the city, across the dry wheat fields, leaving behind a ghostly line between old and new.

PART THREE

☙

NIGHT SWEATS

I wake up cold, I who
Prospered through dreams of heat
Wake to their residue,
Sweat, and a clinging sheet.

—Thom Gunn
The Man with Night Sweats, 1992

❧

Dream Recall

W HAT DOES an insomniac dream? No, this is not an oxymoron. Insomniacs do sleep and do dream, like all other human beings, in spite of our ofttimes vigorous denials in the morning. If Freud's theory about wish fulfillment is right, you'd think we'd dream only of sleep. What could one desire more? I can imagine a recurring dream of lying in my childhood bed or, better yet, in a crib: soft mattress, warm flannel blanket, circus-animal mobile overhead. These elements might be disguised within the dream itself—the slats of the crib as the bars of a cage and so forth. Yet deep within it, smothered under countless layers of symbolism and dreamed-up comforters, lies a clear image of myself, eyes moving under shut lids, soundly sleeping through a full REM cycle.

A lovely fantasy, but in my experience it never comes: the insomniacal mind does not dream of sleep. It would be, I believe, like trying to feed beef to a cow: a form of sleep cannibalism. The fact is, insomniacs dream of the same things that most people dream about: the stuff of everyday life, at once bizarre and prosaic, populated by familiar faces and odd peripheral figures, almost always forgotten upon waking.

I don't even pay much attention to my dreams, unless they feature a celebrity. Joni Mitchell used to make regular appearances when I was a teenager. In a typical dream, we'd sit and talk and she would show me rare bootleg albums of her previously unknown songs; I could see the cover photos and lyric sheets. I'd wake, thinking for a moment these records truly existed, and once even went out and searched for them, fragments of titles still stuck in my head. More recently, I've dreamed of Madonna and Joan Didion, my twin midlife muses, who've granted a few seconds of disposable intimacy. But celebrity dreams, like wet dreams, are exceedingly rare as I get older.

One must cultivate a good dream life to have one, something for which insomniacs such as my friend James seem to be particularly well-suited. He sought my advice several months ago because he was having so much trouble sleeping. (It's ironic how often I have found myself in this position: friends and near strangers consulting me, a failure at sleep, about the best ways to succeed at it. And yet, a lousy athlete may become a great coach—perhaps the same principle applies.)

I could have guessed James was a closet insomniac even before he divulged this piece of information—in the same way it's no surprise when the guy with the pierced tongue, lip, eyebrow, septum, and nostril tells you he had "a bad childhood." At age forty-five, James was what I uncharitably call a "pressed-jean queen," and not only because his Levi's were always crisply ironed. Everything in his presentation was slightly overdetermined, each effect of wardrobe, diet, tanning, and exercise overachieved, every hair in place. He never raised his voice or expressed anger or disappointment—all frustrations were buried until the lights went out. When we sat down in his tiny breakfast nook, I was sure I could smell a faint chemical cloud of sleeping pills wafting from his skin.

"I'm really at the end of my rope," he started. "I can't remember the last time I slept through a night."

At first, I'll admit, my mind was elsewhere. *I could probably count every one of his eyelashes*, I was thinking; *they're so orderly.* I was a little sleep-deprived myself.

"So, what have you tried?" I asked.

"Well, I have a cabinet full of pills."

"Delicious at first, aren't they? You can just relax, place all your trust in them."

"Yeah"—James nodded—"like a new boyfriend."

"And yet, always disappointing. Before you know it, you're back to NyQuil and Tylenol PM. What else have you tried?"

James recited the insomniac's laundry list: massage, acupuncture, herbs, teas, baths, guided visualizations, meditation tapes. Rather than seeing a medical specialist, he had consulted a hypnotherapist. I guess the aura-cleanser didn't have any appointments free. James also mentioned that he kept a dream journal. "Whenever I wake up, I reach for the journal and write down my dreams."

I tried to look intrigued. But, in all honesty, I've never written down my dreams nor been terribly fascinated by others'. A few years ago I bought a book by the novelist Graham Greene, a title I'd never heard of before—excerpts from an eight-hundred-page dream diary he'd kept for twenty-four years. If anyone had fascinating dreams, I thought, he would. Yet within five pages, I knew why it had been on the sale table. Published posthumously, at Greene's request, the book had been given a perfect title, *A World of My Own*. Indeed, it was impenetrable—nicely composed descriptions, yes, but flat, meaningful only to him. And he cut out all the sex. It was like seeing someone's family vacation photos of a generation ago without captions. This is how I feel upon hearing most dreams retold; I had assumed it was a personal quirk, a lack of empathy on my part. But research backs me up: something about dream content itself is inherently forgettable. When put into words, dreams tend to be interesting only to the dreamer.

I asked James how long he had kept a journal. His face lit up: "Oh, it's amazing—ten years of dreams! I've always thought they might provide a key to my insomnia."

I had a hunch and went with it. "Have you ever thought that maybe the journal itself was causing the problem?"

James looked at me, puzzled.

"Maybe you've conditioned yourself *too* well to awaken to your dreams," I said, "to write them down. Do you turn on the light? Sit up? Find your glasses? A pen? And you do this how many times a night? A week?"

As I spoke, James shook his head and groaned.

"Maybe it's time to put the journal away," I offered quietly. "Someplace far from your bedroom."

This impulse to preserve one's dreams, to study and find meaning in them, may have started with our early ancestors. Eighteen thousand years ago, the cave painters at Lascaux recorded their dreams, some experts say. The French neuroscientist Michel Jouvet even speculates that one image at Lascaux shows a Cro-Magnon man in what we'd now call a REM state—he's lying on his back and has a full erection. Surrounded by a bison, a bird, and a broken spear, the cave figure is dreaming of his desire to hunt, Jouvet suggests. (Or simply, I wonder, of his desire to have sex?) Primitive man believed that an invisible "spirit" or "soul" left the body during sleep and wandered freely through space and time, into the past or future.

Clay tablets dating back seven thousand years preserve examples of Babylonian and Assyrian dream interpretations. In ancient religions, from the Egyptians to the Greeks and the Romans, the dreamworld existed outside of waking thought; in dreams, one might receive messages from the gods. Believers slept in special temples, with the hope that the gods would appear to them. In the morning, oracles would explain the dream content. According to Greek mythology, dreams signaled visits from Hypnos' sons: Morpheus, who imitated people; Icelos, who took the form of birds and beasts; and Phantasos, who transformed himself into rocks, water, and other inanimate things. Around 350 B.C., Aristotle wrote the first book in which dreaming was treated as an activity of the mind rather than as a medium for divine communication.

The first modern scholar to systematically study dreaming was a twenty-eight-year-old American, Mary Whiton Calkins, a psychology instructor at Wellesley College. In her influential article "Statistics of Dreams," from the April 1893 *American Journal of Psychology*, she introduced the method of awakening sleepers to collect dreams for the purpose of analysis. Freud owed a debt to Miss Calkins (which he acknowledged), as did Eugene Aserinsky and later researchers. She reported the results of a study in which two "observers," as she called them, were repeatedly awakened by an alarm clock, or of their own volition, to record what they'd seen in their sleep. The first person, Miss Calkins herself, recalled 205 dreams in fifty-five nights; the second, a thirty-two-year-old man identified only as "S," recorded 170 dreams in forty-six nights. I can't help wondering if S was also her research advisor, a man named Sanford, whom she credited, or, perhaps instead, her husband. I love the idea of them waking up in bed together—four times a night, on average—to share ever more wild dream stories.

Miss Calkins categorized and cross-referenced the 375 dreams by type, tone, emotion, setting, "vividness," and time of night, among other measures. While acknowledging that her study was small, she was attempting nothing less than to decode dream logic, to make sense of "the warp and woof of dream experience," and to apply previously unused scientific methods to the process. She concluded—correctly, as later scientists verified—that most dreams occur near dawn and that there's a close relationship between events of the previous day and dream content. (Eighty-nine percent of the dreams had clear connections to the dreamers' waking lives.) Dreams with specific content drew closer study: "word-dreams" were classified by form—was the word spoken, heard, read, or written down?; people in dreams were carefully identified and tabulated—family, friend, well-known, or unknown; the "philosophical character" of dreams was examined; and so on. She made fine distinctions among related dreams and provided keen observations on dream substance.

"We constantly witness in our dreams, without a quaver of surprise, scenes and events of the most wildly improbable character," she wrote. "And just as the dreamer literally does not know enough to be surprised, so also his judgment plays him false in the recognition of the beautiful. I cannot recall a single distinct waking memory of any beautiful dream object, though it is common enough to dream of something as rarely beautiful which one recognizes through the waking recollection as merely fantastic or *bizarre*."

Recalling these ephemeral images and getting them down on paper was a delicate maneuver, Miss Calkins noted. "Sometimes the slight movement of reaching for paper and pencil or of lighting one's candle seems to dissipate the

dream-memory, and one is left with the tantalizing consciousness of having lived through an interesting dream-experience
of which one has not the faintest memory."

Today's researchers call this a white dream, the sleep
state equivalent of a black hole. Some leaders in the field
strongly argue that such an experience is not a dream at all,
that a dream is not "real" until in waking life it can be recounted, which sounds more like a philosophical argument
than a scientific one. (Following this logic, an amnesiac or an
infant could not dream. Nor, for that matter, could a dog.) But
if it is so, if these experts are right, then I propose that the reverse is also true: one's life is not real until he listens to his
dreams. Then, he must fully awaken.

I moved from Seattle to the Castro, as to another country, in
July of 1985, right at the time when Rock Hudson revealed he
had AIDS and every newspaper and magazine was filled with
stories about the deadly epidemic. "Why bother going to San
Francisco?" my father said before I left. He thought I might as
well commit suicide. But I was ecstatic to be at the center of
it all, twenty-four years old and living in a ratty Victorian off
Diamond Street with four roommates, three cats, and a spectacular view of the city.

My college friend David had called a few weeks before
to offer me a vacant room in the flat. Within days, I had quit
my job at Thousand Trails, a membership campground company; given my car to a sister; sold my furniture, stereo, and
books on the sidewalk; and bought a one-way plane ticket, en-
suring that I wouldn't be coming back soon. Still, I left my
record albums with a friend, promising to retrieve them someday. I traded my TV to a neighbor for an astrological chart
reading, but I was in too much of a hurry to have it done. The

air crackled with danger. The community, to which I belonged at last, without question, was fighting for its life. The future was filled with possibilities.

David, who'd recently come out himself, had moved to San Francisco a year before to launch his theater-directing career. He and my new flatmates, Laurie, Paul, and Michael, picked me up at the airport. I was proud that everything I owned could fit into the trunk of his car—two suitcases, a box packed with ten years of journals and poetry, a cassette player, Walkman, and tapes. I had enough cash to last two months, or so I thought: $800.

I already knew San Francisco well, and yet, driving in at dusk, I had never before seen it look so beautiful and strange. When the familiar skyline popped up at the 101/80 split, it appeared that the day's summer heat and light were being choked off by fast-moving fingers of purple fog. By the time we reached Twentieth and Diamond, the night air was chilly and the whole city was under a cloud. To celebrate my arrival, we got drunk on iced vodka while roasting marshmallows over a hibachi on the porch. House lights sparkled from the hills around us, as though sending out SOS signals through the fog.

I inherited a lumpy, stained mattress that had survived several previous flatmates, the last of whom, another college friend, was an actress who'd played the lead in a Santa Clara production of the classical Greek tragedy *Iphigenia in Aulis,* a role she'd never really stopped performing. Iphigenia, as I called her behind her back, had fallen madly in love during the brief time she'd slept on the mattress. As a bridal bouquet is caught by the next-to-wed, would the same good fortune be passed on to me?

Iphigenia had left to move in with her much older boyfriend, a New Age iridologist. It was obvious why they were drawn to one another: Iphigenia had astonishingly beautiful blue-gray eyes that appeared to be stuck open in a lifelong gaze. As for the iridologist, when he wasn't diagnosing the flecks in people's eyes, he was also an aspiring playwright. He had written a play for her, which was closing at a tiny Castro theater the night after I arrived, providing a good excuse to throw another party.

Laurie, with whom I'd gone to school in Florence, was a student at the California Culinary Academy. I helped her cook an extravagant closing-night feast for ten: quail and sausage on the hibachi, homemade pasta, and artichokes. We ate before going to the play, *The Articulation of Andrea*, which was as bad as the title suggests, and then returned to the flat for dessert—flaming plums soaked in cognac—and lines of cocaine. I'd seriously underestimated my share of the food and drug budget.

It was a summer in which I never slept at conventional times, and perhaps for the first time, I didn't care. Sleep schedules were as fluid as house rules. There was always a flatmate to keep me company at most any hour of the night, and we were all usually sleep-deprived. On weekends, daytime drowsiness yielded delicious afternoon naps, a pleasure I hadn't enjoyed before. Sleep was an appetite to be satisfied and experimented with, like sex.

"This is the house of the thousand and one sins," pronounced our friend John—thereby naming our flat—when he paid a visit one Sunday afternoon. He'd stumbled upon the five of us, just out of bed at 3 P.M., sitting in our robes watching a tape of John Waters's *Pink Flamingos*, drinking champagne and eating Laurie's homemade croissants, fresh from the oven but as heavy as bread loaves and as flat as brownies. John accepted a mug of champagne and took a toke on a joint. "Every time I come here, I commit another ghastly sin," he said, raising his cup in a toast.

Many nights during my first months, we'd all go dancing at the Stud, a small Folsom Street bar that seemed to me about as close to heaven as one could get. Not much bigger than our flat, the place was so crowded you had to push your way to the bar for a drink, but it was through a herd of men, which was not unpleasant. Sometimes you'd be almost swept off your feet, as if the doors had opened in a rush-hour subway and you were able to move only with the bodies, not against them. A hand might grab yours, and you'd be led blind, landing safely a few feet away on the dance floor. The music was taped: Bronski Beat giving way to Sade giving way to New Order. Bunches of fresh flowers, votive candles, and old strings of Christmas lights gave the wood-paneled room a funky warmth. Separated at the door from David and the others, I might spot their faces, or the backs of their heads, as I danced and circled the bar, only to meet up again at the end of the night. Having blown all our money on drinks and the cab ride down, we'd walk home at two in the morning—assuming you hadn't found someone to take you home, which was, for us guys, the main reason for going.

Living in the flat meant being involved in David's latest theatrical production, a "performance piece in two movements" titled *Svetlana*. Tracing the life of Joseph Stalin's daughter, it was somehow also about Svetlana's daughter, Olga, and a San Francisco choreographer and her closeted sculptor husband and his gay lover and his jealous boyfriend. We were all still working on the script, music, costumes, and choreography when rehearsals started in the basement of Theatre Rhinoceros, a gay theater in the Mission District. By the time *Svetlana* opened at the end of August for a two-night run, we were calling it an "experimental work-in-progress," a disclaimer that helped explain why it was unintentionally hilarious and incomprehensible.

I was the production's stage manager, which called for a cool head; unlike the cast, I could not get high before the show started. I had to cue the seven actors, while running lights, creating sound effects—a knock on a door, say, before Svetlana was hauled away for interrogation—and shoving various cassette tapes into the sound system. I can still feel the giddy triumph that came with the show's final cues: lights out; boom box on—loud; cast onstage; houselights up; actors bow.

David's wasn't the only artistic venture. Every member of the production also had his or her own dance company or band or writing career—all experimental works-in-progress. I bought a coffee table for a desk at a garage sale; with my mattress as a cushion, I'd sit in my spartan room late at night and think about writing prize-winning poems. But I wasn't depressed enough to write poetry, as I had been in the past, so at first I wrote long letters to my parents and sisters.

I felt I had so much good news to share. Two weeks after arriving, I had gotten a full-time job doing PR for the Eureka Theatre Company, a couple blocks away from Theatre Rhinoceros. I got my first paycheck, about $400, just as my savings ran out. The Eureka, founded on socialist principles, was committed to producing politically and socially conscious theater—Brecht, Dario Fo, Athol Fugard, Caryl Churchill, and a young playwright named Tony Kushner—as I proudly explained to my parents. And, of course, I had to tell them all about *Svetlana*. It was amazing how fast their return letter came. My parents were aghast: now, in their eyes, I was also a Communist sympathizer.

This added insult to injury; my being gay was still a raw wound. When I'd come out to my parents a year before, it was as if I'd shot them each in the back and the bullet could never safely be removed. Instinctively, they thought I was the one who needed help—a sick child. They felt that I should immediately move back home from Seattle. I declined, only to find a Catholic priest at my door a short time later, sent over from Spokane by my parents like a messenger from God. He counseled that I could *be* gay without being sexually active. "Oh,

I've tried that already," I replied. As a compromise, I agreed to see a psychiatrist in Seattle, both individually and, when they made trips to Seattle, with Mom and Dad. In our first "family session" after I'd seen him several times, the psychiatrist reported that I was remarkably well-adjusted. Perhaps my parents could benefit from some private therapy? My father stormed out, angry as hell.

In San Francisco, I came to dread the sight of his handwriting on an envelope, his worried and admonishing voice on the phone. Following family tradition, I went to Spokane that first Christmas, yet it seemed as if we never stopped arguing—whether about my job, my "lifestyle," my finances, my clothes. I was naive enough at the time to think that they should be happy for me. But, to them, I had become unlike any person they'd known—someone so far from who they were that little still bound us. When I left on New Year's Eve, I could just as easily have been stepping off the face of the earth as returning to Gay Mecca. And, in fact, I didn't return to Spokane for nine years.

My father had actually lived in San Francisco for several months at about the same age I was then. After being wounded in the war, he was flown to the Bay Area and hospitalized at the Presidio, a beautiful military compound on a hill dotted with redwoods, right near the Golden Gate Bridge. None of which he could see—both his eyes were covered with bandages for many weeks. I can only imagine his terror: Having barely made it alive out of Korea, he was confined to a hospital bed, blind, in a city he didn't know, without family or friends nearby. His distinguished and exciting military career, as he'd planned it since he was a young man, was over. What was he going to do with his life?

When he was well enough, Dad once told me, he'd leave Letterman Hospital at night (a patch over his blind eye) to go to the jazz clubs in North Beach. This was the early 1950s—

San Francisco in its boho-beatnik days—and the places must have been hopping. Dad had played drums for years, once formed a trio with his brother and a friend, and dreamed of being a jazz musician. I can't help wondering if he might have been tempted, at that moment in his life, to go for it. He'd dismiss the idea if I asked him about it today. But I can almost see him, at age twenty-six, his head bopping to the music as he sips a Scotch in a smoky club: he's thinking about it, he's thinking about it. He tips the waitress, who won't let a soldier pay for a drink, then spends the night wandering through San Francisco.

My father would never have recognized the city that I called home. I lived in a gay neighborhood that did not exist thirty years before. I belonged to a gay gym. I shopped at a grocery store, Cala Foods, where not only were all the clerks gay or lesbian, but almost all the customers. Buying cigarettes or a quart of milk at 4 A.M., one might also pick up someone in the express line to take home.

Not that one's opportunities ended at the store. In the Castro, shadows came to life at night, like figments of a child's imagination—a child who is not afraid of, but enraptured by, the dark. I can see myself walking up Eighteenth Street in the middle of the night. I glance up: there, on the third floor of that Victorian, a naked man appears in the window. I stop to look but in a blink he's gone. There's only the slightest breeze; it is as though I can feel and hear people drawing breath. If I stare into the dark with enough concentration, I can make out figures all around me—men in windows, inside cars, in the bushes in Collingwood Park. I can hear them whispering, moaning. They're there and not there, gone in a flash, like targets in a carnival shooting gallery.

The neighborhood was fed by these images, made more intensely alive by them. Darkness hid signs of illness, turning a ravaged city into a tense erotic dreamscape, and infected bodies into unblemished ones. With daylight, signs of the nightmare emerged. My first deep sense of foreboding came not in a blunt way but indirectly, in the disappearance of men I did not know. Someone I would commonly see at the gym or on the bus or at Cala Foods, or a man I would purposefully look for at the Stud, returning week after week and hoping to meet him, was suddenly missing. He could have moved to another neighborhood or city, received a job transfer, or joined a new gym. He could have been hit by a bus, I would remind myself, finding a measure of comfort in such violent accidents. But I soon learned that the lottery-logic spun to answer such questions in most people's lives held little currency here.

Terribly familiar with illness, some men I knew seemed able to spot it from blocks away, even in the earliest stages—and this was before the HIV antibody test provided absolute proof. It was "that look," they called it, as though talking about changing weather—a drop in barometric pressure before a bad storm.

Faces of the dead surfaced weekly, reappearing after several months or years missing as small black-and-white snapshots in the *Bay Area Reporter*, a local gay newspaper, which published the latest obituaries. Picking up a copy, I habitually opened first to this section. Some weeks, there were only a handful of faces. Other times, they crowded two pages or more. After a year in San Francisco, I always recognized someone I'd known casually—danced, slept, or worked out with. In a macabre twist, it became spookier to spot someone on the street alive, whom I had assumed already to be dead, than to realize another man was missing.

After scanning the photographs, I started at the top again and read the birth dates, stopping to read the obituaries of men who were my age or younger when they'd died—1961, 1963, 1970. Haunted by my own good fortune, I was seized by a particular queasiness. I knew that, in a barely different scenario, it could have been me.

In nightmares, it *was* me: I had AIDS, my body oozing with sores, skin melting. Jarred awake by such dreams, I trained myself to snuff them out with a technique I still use. I'd pounce on a preset mental image or idea, such as *What does water taste like?* while picturing a tall, clear glass in hand. I'd focus on the water's coolness and keep drinking until the nightmares faded. I tried turning them into "white dreams," in essence.

Maybe this is precisely *why* some nightmares recur, it strikes me now—the forced effort to disremember never allows them to defuse—never to burn to the end of the wick, sputter, then die out. It's a theory I'd like to have run by Eugene Aserinsky, especially knowing that a hair-raisingly bad dream had played a small but key role in his early REM research. The incident had occurred late one evening in the University of Chicago's sleep lab. A young man under observation was in the midst of a "REM hurricane" that almost unhinged the pens on the lab equipment, Aserinsky first noticed. He rushed to the sleeping subject's bedside and called his name.

Upon waking, the man asked, "Was I having a nightmare?" almost like a child seeking reassurance from his dad— *There, there, it was only a dream. Go back to sleep.* But Aserinsky didn't placate; he asked the man to describe it in detail. It was the sort he often had while at home, the subject explained, in which he feared that he'd never wake up and would die in his sleep. Aserinsky couldn't have been happier. He knew at once that the subject's nightmare and the wild REM tracing were related. Following the tests with his own son and the botched experiment with the blind student, this was Aserinsky's most powerful early evidence that REM was linked to dreaming.

You'd think that Aserinsky would then have pestered the subject with questions: What was this dream death like? Did you know you were dreaming *in* the dream? To Aserinsky, though, the significant fact was that the subject could *recall* his nightmare. Its content, source, or potential meaning was inconsequential. Aserinsky was interested in dreaming as a physiological event rather than as a tool for understanding human behavior. In fact, he was skeptical of therapeutic dream analysis—"Freudian falderal," he called it—which later struck his son, Armond, as ironic.

"As part of my own training as a psychiatrist, I've been through fairly extensive psychoanalytic therapy," Armond told me. "And one thing I had great trouble with was talking about my dreams. I would just bristle when the analyst would ask me about them. It would cause an instant transference reaction. At that point, it would be like talking to my father. I'd have to remind the analyst, 'You know, you're talking to the son of REM.'"

His father's anti-Freudian, reductionist view of dreaming was in agreement with Nathaniel Kleitman's. "To those who insist that because dreams occur they must serve a particular purpose, it may be pointed out that not all processes have a teleological explanation," he wrote in *Sleep and Wakefulness*. To illustrate his point, he offered a typically Kleitmanian analogy: vomiting. "When it is elicited by some irritating matter in the stomach . . . [vomiting] serves a good purpose in evacuating the stomach and removing the irritant. The same vomiting act, when resulting from motion sickness, serves no physiological purpose." So, too, with dreaming, in Dr. Kleitman's opinion: it may be as biologically meaningless as getting carsick.

Under Dr. Kleitman's supervision, William C. Dement took up the REM research where Aserinsky left off when he moved to Seattle. At this early point in his career, Dement has written, he was fascinated by dreaming; he was even planning to become a psychoanalyst. In studies at the University of Chicago laboratory involving over three hundred subjects, he and Dr. Kleitman confirmed in 1957 that dreams are most likely to occur during REM sleep. This was used as a definitive criterion in subsequent research: If REM sleep is the dream state, then one awakens the subject from REM to retrieve a dream. Failure to report a dream was considered a failure to recall.

Now we know, of course, that dreams may occur in both REM and NREM sleep—or they may not. At least 17 percent of a REM cycle, for instance, is dreamless. Further, whether or not one *recalls* a dream is incidental, some researchers say. Which is not the same as suggesting that dreaming is pointless (as still others contend). On the contrary. Scientists such as Avi Karni and Dov Sagi at Israel's Weismann Institute believe that REM sleep is crucial for consolidating memories. It operates, they have proposed, like a computer program that organizes and cleans up all of one's disparate files. Dreaming is a glimpse at memories as they're being put into different areas of brain storage. Other scientists are less convinced of REM's memory-consolidating role. Francis Crick, one of the Nobel laureates who discovered the structure of DNA, takes the opposite view. He, along with Graeme Mitchison and others, has proposed that REM sleep disposes of unneeded memories. Dreaming is a last glance at the trash as its being tossed out.

The difference between the two views sounds to me like the classic argument of perception: Is the glass half-empty or half-full? Perhaps there is no single right way to look at it. Maybe dreaming is a neuropsychological function that is adaptable, depending on the circumstances of the day, and the events over a period of time. Some nights we dream to remember our lives. Some nights we dream to forget.

But are there things one *never* dreams about? After analyzing hundreds of dreams from every conceivable perspective, Mary Whiton Calkins stepped back from her work over a century ago and asked herself this question. What was missing from dream life? She came up with a single category: "In times of bereavement, one seldom dreams of the dead." Miss Calkins confirmed her hunch first by searching the dream records used in her study; she and S had lost a mutual friend during that period, yet this person never appeared in a dream.

She also consulted with colleagues. The French scientist Ives Délage told her that during a long period of deep sorrow, he, too, never once dreamed of the friend he had lost, "though he tried to provoke such dreams," a gesture I find extremely touching. What did he try? I wonder. Looking through a photo album before sleep? Reading old letters? Silently invoking his friend's name in the dark? Such efforts are futile, Miss Calkins believed, because the emotions associated with a recently deceased loved one are too overwhelming and complex. I agree. It's as though the dreaming mind protects the mourning body so it can rest. Conjuring up ghosts is properly left for daydreaming—or night terrors. But later, much later, one may often dream of the dead. It happens, I've found, only once your most vivid memories have faded, years after grief has passed.

Billy's boyfriend, Gary, was the first person I knew well to go. He died while sitting in a chair in their apartment at dinnertime. He'd just eaten half a sandwich, I remember Billy telling me, and then he closed his eyes. He didn't make a sound. How strange and horrible, I thought, that your life could end like that: stopped, without a word. Billy kept waiting for him to wake up.

I had met Gary and Billy through my first serious boyfriend, Nick, with whom I had started living in June of 1986. A year and a half later, we were helping to take care of Peter, one of our closest friends, having already seen Eugene and others die of AIDS. Every time one life ended, another friend started to get really sick.

Peter, a darling and fastidious twenty-nine-year-old from Germany, managed every detail of his treatment and care. One evening in April of 1988, he called a meeting in his bedroom for everyone who'd been helping him out over the past months—bringing in food, cleaning, driving him to the doctor. Eight or ten of us stood around the bed. As Peter began speaking, I watched his hands, the only parts of his body not mottled with black and purple KS lesions.

"If you've seen me over the past weeks since I came home from the hospital, you know that every day I have a little decline," he said. "I had hoped that things would get better, but I know there's not going to be a reverse. I'm going to die soon." He spoke so calmly, rationally, as if scripted for a movie, and yet it could not have been more *like* Peter, or more real. "This morning, I was sitting in the bathtub—after struggling for such a long time just to get into it before the water turned cold—and I was thinking about it, about dying soon, and I started smiling. I don't know—maybe tomorrow I'll be screaming and hysterical, but right now I'm looking forward to it."

He had instructions for each of us: who would help him bathe; who'd help him with bowel movements; who would make arrangements with the Neptune Society for his cremation. "I want you to know that there will be some hard times, and if you're not comfortable with it, that's okay. I mean, I'm fine now, I'm alert, but soon I might not be. I've told my doctor that I'm going to stop taking all the pills on Wednesday. If you're here with me alone and I go into a coma, don't call an ambulance. I don't want people coming in here and putting me on a respirator. I don't want to go to the hospital." He died twelve days later, exactly as he had planned: in bed, lulled to sleep by a large dose of morphine in warm milk. As he requested, I wrote his obituary for the *Bay Area Reporter*.

Shortly after Peter's death, I visited Jeff in the hospital. About my age, Jeff had led a ragged, aimless life. After a stint in the navy, he had moved to the city, where he bounced from job to job, busing tables and bartending. He was as sweet-tempered, impulsive, and endearing as a child—and just as fearful, needy, and helpless when he didn't feel well. Jeff possessed neither the stomach nor the aptitude to become "a model PWA," as Peter had, living with AIDS stoically. Jeff didn't have much money. He had no relatives in San Francisco. No lover, no ex-lover, just a scattering of fuck-buddies and a few casual friends, such as Nick and me. Yet not knowing Jeff well allowed me a different perspective. Against his sketchy life, the disease itself surfaced in monstrous relief.

He was smiling pleasantly when I walked into his hospital room. His face was tilted up at the television; the sound was loud; he did not hear me come in. In the blue light, he had the opaline skin of an infant. His eyes were beautifully large, watery, and still. I sat by his bed and asked how he was doing. "They've got me on morphine. A pill every eight hours. I love it," he said. "I can't feel anything." Absentmindedly, Jeff pushed the thin cotton gown off his shoulder to scratch his arm. His collarbone looked like a rake claw piercing his chest.

He had staged a suicide attempt in his doctor's waiting room so that he would be quickly admitted to the hospital. He called first to tell the receptionist that he was in horrible pain from one of his headaches, weak from diarrhea, and that he wanted just to go to the hospital, but she said he would have to come into the office first to be examined. It would be a four-hour wait.

"I took just enough to faint—only pills," Jeff explained.

"You have to take more—and alcohol—to do it all the way." He knew what he was talking about: he had sent away for information on dosages from the Hemlock Society after he was diagnosed with AIDS. He had traded a friend some AZT for some Seconal.

"I don't know, I guess I'm not ready to check out yet," Jeff said. "I just wanted to stay here for a while—my roommate was being an asshole. Didn't really count on all of this, though. Now they've got me on an IV and a social worker parked at my door." He glanced at the empty chair. "She's a bitch. She just sits there all day long, knitting or chewing gum or talking. I can't even walk outside. She must be off taking a piss, or the two of you would be best friends by now."

A nurse interrupted. Jeff took his eyes off the television and pushed himself up in bed as a tray of food was placed in front of him. "I'm on a liquid diet," he explained. "This is juice, bouillon, Jell-O. I'm not going to eat the ice cream." Every movement, every word, was slowed down, deliberate, graceful, as if he were underwater.

He traced the top of the plastic teacup with a finger. "The biggest dick I ever saw was this thick," he said, suddenly smiling, looking up at me. "And it was this long." He held his hands about a foot apart. "It was the biggest cock I ever saw in my life." Jeff savored the image, giggling softly.

After his release from the hospital, Jeff stayed with Stuart, whom he had met several years earlier at a Dope-Enders meeting. Stuart had ARC (AIDS-related complex, a diagnostic limbo before "full-blown AIDS") and was in the sixth week of a hunger strike to protest the meager federal and state AIDS budget. Hunger strikes, however, weren't attracting a lot of media attention at the time. After years of ignorance and denial, the major newspapers and television news stations were striving to present "positive portraits" of People Living With AIDS, a category Stuart didn't neatly fall into. While his cause was taken up by the gay press, elected officials ignored Stuart and his letter-writing campaign. And it was difficult, even for much of the gay community, to show sympathy for such a grim, fanatical person. Stuart was someone who you thought really would starve himself to death.

I visited his tiny Castro apartment on a cold night to bring Jeff some food. Opening the front door was like cracking open an oven turned to three hundred fifty degrees. I immediately began unpeeling layers of clothing. Stuart was propped on the couch, wrapped in a sleeping bag, shivering, between two plump older men. With his blond hair, emaciated face, and wire-rim glasses, he looked like a medicated Pilgrim.

The room was lit by a collection of seven or eight electric space heaters that crackled, hissed, and wheezed, bursting on and off, and cast a warm orange glow on the floor. It was as though I had wandered into an infernal chapel. No one spoke a word. The door had disappeared behind me. The only thing on the wall was a giant calendar covered with X's, marking Stuart's countdown.

"Jeff's sleeping," one of the men finally said. "Do you want to sit down?"

Standing there, I felt for one delirious moment the true terror of illness: being horribly, inescapably trapped, just like Jeff and Stuart—trapped *in* life, in a body that refuses to die, and desperate to break free of it. I thought, if I join the other two men quietly waiting their turn on the couch, if I make myself at home here, I will never leave this apartment.

I found my way to the kitchen, placed the food in the empty refrigerator, then looked in on Jeff. The last image I have of him alive is in that dim, hothouse bedroom. In spite of the heat, he was sprawled diagonally atop the bed, facedown, wearing a hat, gloves, and a winter coat, as if he had fallen in knee-high snow and couldn't get himself up again.

A couple days later, Stuart found Jeff dragging a bucket of water and a space heater around the apartment, searching for an electric socket. Jeff had to go back into the hospital—the psychiatric ward, this time—where he was forced to participate in group therapy and undergo a battery of neurological tests. The doctors could not find anything wrong with him.

Jeff stopped talking after several days in the ward, I was told. I remember thinking, I'm not surprised: this shy and gentle kid is ready to die, and he doesn't want to talk about it to anyone—whether doctor, social worker, or friend—anymore. I interpreted his silence as a noble surrender. "Jeff passed on, at peace and without fear," his obituary would begin. It wasn't until he died a few weeks later and an autopsy was performed that doctors finally discovered lesions on Jeff's brain, due to AIDS, which had caused his dementia and loss of speech.

Chapter 14

⤳

Hypnotics

I WAKE AND think of sleep. *I've done it:* that's my first thought. Having hit the snooze button, my few final minutes of bed warmth are made more marvelous by this sense of accomplishment. Dream images tease memory as my brain waves shift into full alpha; eyes shut, I permit myself to count the hours: *Fell asleep about midnight, subtract thirty minutes for the 3 A.M. pee and some back-in-bed restlessness. Okay, that's six solid hours. Good job.* I turn off the alarm. But as I shuffle into the kitchen to make coffee, I begin thinking about the moment eighteen hours from now when I'll turn the alarm on and the reading light off. Pride and relief are drained and replaced by a fresh thought: *Can I do it again?*

This obsessive daily dose of self-doubt may be the single

characteristic that separates natural-born insomniacs from all others. Even when we've slept well, we suspect it may be the last such episode. Every night's a new story. We're like mountain gorillas whose days are spent in search of another leafy tree to eat from, a sheltered clearing to nest in, safe from predators. At dawn we cover our tracks and set out to find a way to get back to sleep come nightfall.

I would love to see how gorillas do it; observe them in the wild. An inability to sleep outdoors, however, immediately disqualifies me. I couldn't even fall asleep in my own backyard when I was a boy. Some nights, though, I do camp out in front of the TV. I long for the magic remote that would let me skip through the decades, not just the channels. In 1955, there was a live TV show for insomniacs called *Count Sheep* that aired nightly in the New York area right after NBC's *Tonight* show. Featuring a pretty, twenty-nine-year-old model, Nancy Berg, dressed in a long, frilly nightgown, it followed her through a soothing bedtime routine of cuddling a cocker spaniel, reading aloud in bed, then saying good-night with a yawn and a stretch. The half-hour show closed with a graphic of fence-jumping sheep, recalls Berg, who's now retired and living in New York City. "At that time I knew little about sleep," she told me with a gust of laughter, "since I was taking amphetamines in an effort to be model-thin. I didn't sleep for about ten years."

Though it sounds as if it was designed for straight male viewers, I'd kill to see reruns of *Count Sheep* at 1 A.M. At that hour, most TV shows, and especially the commercials, are too loud and frenetic to be relaxing. I'm a sucker for those dull, plodding educational programs about wild animals. Not the juiced-up ones featuring celebrities—*The Elephants of India with Goldie Hawn*. But the real deal: where the animals have far more personality than the zoologists and primatologists; the program is scored with corny music; and the off-camera commentator seems to be the same deep-voiced man who narrated public-school films in the late sixties. Thank God for cable TV. I can find one of these shows on at almost any time of the night. With their slow pace and long stretches of complete silence—a wide shot of the veld, say, as vultures rip apart a gazelle carcass—they have a soporific quality that makes them transfixing to insomniacs.

Of course, they are not without drama. Few things are more thrilling than watching an enormous and powerful animal subdued by humans—an elephant saved from ivory poachers, for example, by sedating and transporting it to a game preserve. The park rangers are positioned right in front of the cameraman, whispering their strategy, tranquilizer rifles hoisted: *Okay, now we'll aim for the back left flank. Won't feel a thing.* Poing! The dart finds its target, blooms, and in seconds, a five-ton elephant stumbles to the ground.

I would like to *be* that elephant, I think some nights—knocked out cold. What's in those tranquilizers? Write me a prescription, Jack Hanna. Maybe I could boil it down, chop it up, and put it into capsules. Or I could buy a tranquilizer rifle for Steve—one with a silencer. He'd aim for the birthmark on my ass and shoot me as I go to take a pee after lying awake for three hours. Ah, bliss: felled right on the bathroom rug.

Instead, I turn off the TV, go to the kitchen, and rummage for the bottle of Ambien in the pill cabinet. Ambien is the brand name for zolpidem tartrate, a short-acting "hypnotic" (as sleeping pills are called). At present, it's the most widely prescribed sleeping pill in the world. Ambien is one of several new drugs called nonbenzodiazepine hypnotics, which are rapidly absorbed and quickly eliminated from the body. This makes them useful for people who have trouble initially falling asleep. Their sedative effect lasts no more than four hours, reducing groggy drug hangovers. Nonbenzodiazepines have recently been developed with an even lighter sedative ef-

fect than Ambien. There's one named Sonata—how lyrical!—
that can safely be taken in the middle of the night just to help
a person fall back asleep.

For those who awaken frequently, a physician may prescribe a drug with a heavier sedative effect, such as Restoril,
from another class of hypnotics, benzodiazepines. While Ambien is not related chemically to Restoril, their action is similar. Both are thought to modulate a neurotransmitter in the
brain, the GABA receptor. Beyond that, however, scientists
cannot say with absolute certainty how these and other hypnotics work. A third group of sleeping pills, barbiturates, includes highly addictive sedatives such as Seconal and Nembu-
tal; these are recommended only for people with extreme
difficulty sleeping, perhaps due to pain from serious illness or
injury. While sleeping pills facilitate sleep, they can also
change its structure. Barbiturates exert a long-lasting sedative
effect, for example, yet decrease REM sleep and the deep,
restful sleep of stages 3 and 4. After eight hours' sleep, a person may wake still feeling tired. By contrast, drugs such as
Ambien and Restoril generally do not interfere with normal
sleep stages.

I've been using Ambien on bad nights, two or three times
a month, for a couple of years, and it works well, yet I still feel
as if I'm doing something dishonest. I am, technically: my prescription expired long ago, so I steal from Steve's. (I usually
confess the next morning.) He keeps it at the back of the pill
shelf in the corner, where it belongs, I believe—there being a
moral hierarchy for prescription drugs. All of Steve's meds are
stationed right up front—the ones he takes daily. Vitamins,
herbs, and aspirin occupy the middle ground, a neutral zone in
advance of the sleeping pills, antacids, antinausea pills, and
decongestants. It's not that sleeping pills are bad per se, but
there is something disreputable about them. I wouldn't want
the Ambien bottle to accidentally fall out of the cabinet in

front of the pest-control man. Nor should it be very easy to reach. One should always have to find a sleeping pill, go to a little trouble. The decision to take one should not be taken lightly. Its rewards are too valuable.

An ex-junkie once told me that the sight of a syringe—even a photograph—still gave him an intense physical craving to shoot up. I know, in part, what he means: sometimes just holding the amber-colored bottle of Ambien in my hand is enough to make me drowsy. I'm always surprised by how large the container is for so few pills—just thirty per prescription, and Steve has broken them all in half for an even lighter dose. I pour them onto my palm: with their craggy edges and polished white surfaces, the Ambiens look like a small pile of tooth fragments. Not human teeth but an ocean creature's, such as the Indus dolphin of the Arabian Sea, which actually sleeps seven hours a day while swimming. From the mouth of a dolphin, I imagine, to my own: I pick out a big chip and put it on my tongue. I let it dissolve for a moment—believing this will speed up the effect—taste its bitterness, and swallow.

While humans have likely been doping themselves to sleep since the earliest days as hunter-gatherers, the ancient Greeks were among the first to record their remedies. Greek physicians made a hypnotic compound from poppy seeds, the raw source for the narcotic morphine (named after Morpheus, god of dreams). According to ancient medical texts, numerous plants were used in gentler sleep elixirs, from lettuce leaves to chamomile flowers. Edward Binns, M.D., author of *The Anatomy of Sleep*, dated the first use of hypnotics further back, to the royal courts of ancient Egypt and the Far East. "By the glare of torches, night had been turned into day, to prolong the revels of a favorite sultana" or to gratify other "libidinous whims," he wrote in 1842, "for wealth had acquired the art of contracting the enjoyments of a life-time within the circle of an evening. It therefore required new soporifics, and powerful narcotics, to procure rest," such as palm wine, which he claimed was also used to preserve the dead. During the Middle Ages, others have noted, those who had difficulty sleeping would suck on a swab soaked in a potent cocktail of poppy extract and alcohol. The poppy was used in its purer form, opium, as a treatment for insomnia through the nineteenth century.

One of the first American physicians to make a clinical specialty of treating insomnia was William Alexander Hammond, who had a thriving practice in New York in the late 1800s. Dr. Hammond, who started out as a medical officer stationed in Kansas prior to the Civil War, had developed a novel theory of sleep after observing in 1854 a patient who'd suffered a terrible skull fracture. In a railroad accident, the man had lost a three-by-six-inch portion of his skull. Dr. Hammond noticed that the scalp—presumably stitched back into place over the fissure—sank slightly during sleep and returned to the level of the cranium when the man was awake. Hammond later made similar observations of sleeping newborns with unclosed "soft spots" (fontanels) and conducted research on dogs and rabbits that convinced him his theory was correct. In an 1865 article, "On Sleep and Insomnia," Dr. Hammond announced his finding to the medical community: sleep was caused by a decrease in blood in the brain, "cerebral anemia," a conclusion that contradicted the prevailing view that sleep resulted from vascular *congestion* of the brain. Insomnia, he deduced, was therefore caused by an excess of blood in the brain, a neurological disease he called cerebral hyperaemia.

Modern science has long since disproved Hammond's theory: yes, a rise and fall in brain pressure does occur, but it has no bearing on wakefulness or sleep. In his day, nevertheless, he thought he'd made a critical breakthrough. Dr. Hammond spread his views on sleep through articles written for both medical journals and popular magazines of the day, and through a series of books, including a memoir and thinly veiled scientific novels. He was the Michael Crichton of the late-Victorian era, in my conception: tall, dashing, rich, prolific. He knew how to tell a good story. An article on the dangers of unwanted "wakefulness" (as insomnia was also known) written for *Appleton's Journal,* for instance, opened with a cautionary tale he'd learned from a foreign colleague. It concerned a Chinese merchant who had been convicted of murdering his wife. "The judges determined to punish him in such a manner as to inflict the utmost amount of suffering," Dr. Hammond wrote, "and, at the same time, strike terror into the hearts of all those who might entertain the idea of following his example. He was, accordingly, condemned to die by being deprived of sleep."

Guarded round the clock by three policemen, the prisoner was given food and drink but prevented from falling asleep. "At first the condemned man congratulated himself on the mildness of his punishment, and was rather disposed to regard the whole matter as a joke," Dr. Hammond continued. "By the third day, however, he began to feel very uncomfortable. His eyes were red, his mouth parched, his skin dry and hot, and his head ached." By the eighth day, in brief moments of lucidity, the killer begged authorities to end his torture. "He implored them to grant him the blessed opportunity of being strangled, guillotined, burned to death, drowned, garroted, shot, quartered, blown up with gunpowder, cut into small pieces, or killed in any conceivable way their humanity or ferocity might suggest." All was in vain—his captors coolly turned a deaf ear.

By this point, the prisoner couldn't have slept even if allowed, Dr. Hammond explained, inserting his own theories into the tale: "The brain was feeding on the products of its own disintegration, and sleep was impossible. He was now entirely insane." Insanity was inevitable, the doctor believed, because, without rest, the brain was self-destructing, unable to replenish itself. "Finally, nature gave way altogether." On the nineteenth day, "death released him from his sufferings."

Lack of sleep certainly wasn't the killer's killer but was a likely contributor. Regardless of the actual cause of death, the Chinese prisoner's story must have helped stir up business. Fearing a similar fate, insomniacs flocked to Dr. Hammond for a cure. By the late 1860s, according to the medical historian Bonnie Ellen Blustein, his New York practice was highly successful and he had achieved international renown. For a quarter of a century, he treated thousands of people for cerebral hyperaemia, among other neurological ailments. In general practice, Dr. Hammond believed that hyperaemia could be caused by intensive study, excessive work, or strong emotion. People who "overused their brains," such as inventors, female students, and Wall Street speculators, were most likely to become victims of the disease, with insomnia being one of its earliest symptoms.

In his book *On Wakefulness,* Dr. Hammond described a typical case: "A gentleman, aged thirty-nine, unmarried, of correct habits, and good general health, consulted me on the 19th of April, 1865, in reference to a peculiar nervous affection with which he had suffered for several months. He stated to me that, being engaged upon a literary labor of some importance, he had given the greater part of his time to the studies necessary to its being carried on with success, and was conscious of having overtasked his mental powers. So great, however, was his ambition to excel in his undertaking, that he had persevered notwithstanding the admonitions of friends, and the still more pointed warnings he had received from his own sensations." Instead of sleeping eight hours, he frequently slept less than four out of twenty-four.

I daresay Dr. Hammond could have been describing *me*, or perhaps a vaguely related ancestor. In a note to the doctor, the unmarried gentleman gave permission to use his experience as a case study. "I make only one condition," he wrote. "You know I am a literary man, and that my reputation as a student and author would suffer in the estimation of the critics were I suspected of insanity. It takes very little to form a foundation for such an assumption, and, perhaps, in my case, there would be more truth than fiction in the notion as applied to me. With the exception, therefore, of giving my name, you are at perfect liberty to dish me up for the satisfaction of all your medical friends."

Dish he did. "His bowels, contrary to what might have been reasonably expected, were regular, and his appetite was generally good," Dr. Hammond reported. More troubling than the loss of sleep to the patient was the loss of clarity in his writing, the subject of which was Greek drama. At the end of the day, he often found that he had written the exact opposite of what he'd intended. "I was confident that his condition was clearly the result of intense hyperaemia of the brain," Dr. Hammond noted, "and that if this could be dissipated, and sound, regular, and sufficient sleep be produced, the mental trouble would also vanish."

To reduce the excessive blood in his brain, the Literary Man would have to follow Dr. Hammond's strict orders: Every evening was to include a warm bath. While in the bath, cold water should be poured on his head. Instead of lying down when ready to sleep, he was advised to sit in a chair, with his head on a "hair pillow." All mental labor was to cease. He was only to read novels, no tragedies. Bedtime was set at 11 P.M.

More a vacation than a prescription, Dr. Hammond's

elaborate cure also governed daytime activity. The Literary Man was to rise at seven, "take his sponge bath as usual, and, after eating a moderate breakfast, to do anything he liked, except studying or writing, till twelve o'clock, when he was to take a walk for an hour, then eat a biscuit, read light literature till four, and then ride on horseback till six, at which hour he was to dine, simply, but to the extent his appetite prompted him. He had been in the habit of smoking one cigar a day (after dinner), and I allowed him to continue in this indulgence."

If the gentleman followed this regimen, Dr. Hammond was certain he would not need to resort to bloodletting or to medicinal agents. For the latter, the doctor employed opium on rare occasions. His usual remedy of choice was potassium bromide combined with digitalis, pepsin, and charcoal. This "inky black mixture," historian Blustein has noted, became Dr. Hammond's trademark. Exactly how it was consumed, I do not know (by the spoonful, stirred in water, I'd guess); however, it must have been vile. The bromide was the same compound used in making photographic paper.

In this case, the patient never had to try it. Dr. Hammond's "hygienic regimen" did the trick, it seems: the man pronounced himself cured in a note of thanks. "I would stand on my head with joy, were it not that you were desirous of keeping as much blood out of my noddle as possible," he wrote. *"Laus Deo.* Can I go to work Monday?"

❧

One hundred twenty-three years later, I was the unmarried gentleman seated in a doctor's waiting room seeking a first-time cure for my insomnia. Unmarried but attached: age twenty-seven, I had been referred to Charlie Williamson by my boyfriend, Nick. Dr. Williamson was not a neurologist or sleep specialist but a general practitioner with an office a couple blocks from our apartment near the Castro. A middle-aged gay man with a soft Southern drawl, he had a mustache and thick, wiry hair the color of a rain cloud. Over a few years, his practice had become, by default, almost exclusively devoted to AIDS. But, unlike every other young man in the waiting room, that wasn't one of my concerns: repeated tests over the past two years had confirmed, to my profound surprise and relief, that I was, like Nick, HIV-negative.

Dr. Williamson did an exam and found me in good health. I was sheepish when I explained why I'd come to see him. "Are you kidding?" he responded with a laugh. "Don't apologize. You can't imagine how nice it is to treat something that actually can *be* treated." Then he added, "I've got something for you; I use it myself." He gave me a prescription for a popular benzodiazepine: Halcion.

The only other time I'd taken a sleeping pill was at age twenty, when I'd checked myself into the college infirmary with a long-running flu. I didn't ask for one, it was given to me—standard practice, I suppose; it was probably easier on the clinic's night nurse just to put everyone to sleep. It was definitely a long-lasting drug, perhaps something in the barbiturate family, such as Seconal. When I woke late the next morning, I felt stuck to the bed, as though my flesh had been caramelized.

Since then, I'd suffered melodramatically through my sleepless nights, huffing in frustration as I tossed. After coming out, I rarely stayed overnight when I had sex with someone. Gazing at their boyish sleeping faces in the muddy light was pleasurable for ten minutes, then I started to hate them. More than cuddling, I genuinely liked the cab ride or walk home alone at 2 A.M.; the one-night stand trimmed to its cold, skinny core. I felt in complete possession of myself, of what I wanted to do, as never before. I became expert at kicking a date out of my own bed and, like a true passive-aggressive, making it seem like his decision. "You can stay, if you'd like, but you know, I do have to get up at six," I'd fib. "It might be easier to get a taxi now."

With Nick, who was eleven years older than me, that I didn't want to leave his bed was a first sign of love. It later became a test of it: my sleeplessness often kept Nick awake as well. My insomnia was not more frequent than in the past, but sharing a bed with someone who slept well, it became much more noticeable. Sometimes I left the bed to medicate myself with a glass of red wine, which calmed my nerves but didn't help me sleep. For a time, I took tablets of L-tryptophan, the amino acid found in roast turkey that causes post-Thanksgiving-dinner lethargy. But the tablets were banned by the FDA in 1989 when they were associated with a serious illness, eosinophilia-myalgia syndrome, and at least thirty-eight deaths—something I found hard to believe. Even in combination with other over-the-counter sedatives, such as Sleep-Eze, L-tryptophan had had little impact on me. Now, I was grateful to have something guaranteed to work. *Halcion*: I liked the sound of it, its deliberate evocation of "halcyon days," of happiness and tranquillity. The .25-milligram pill, the highest recommended dose, was colored powder blue, like both a clear sky and the bottom of a swimming pool.

At first, it knocked me out so thoroughly as to leave behind just one residual effect: I remembered nothing. Sleep became an absence, like a long mathematical equation in negative numbers—something my brain could not conceive. I couldn't count the hours because I didn't know exactly when they had started. Nothing happened to remember sleep *by*— no awakenings, no dreams, no getting up to pee. My morning self-doubt about whether I would get back to sleep at night also disappeared for a while. The next day's drug hangover was no worse than insomnia's fatigue. But with each refill of Halcion, I became more tolerant and the benefits dissipated—a typical reaction to any hypnotic. One sleeping pill alone soon failed to put me right to sleep.

I'd lie in bed hyperconscious of my body: heart pounding, blood rushing, chest hairs bristling, skin itching, eyes burning. It reminded me of taking psilocybin mushrooms in college, something I'd done enthusiastically six or seven times until I had a bad trip. Wired on Halcion, I sometimes had a similar panicky feeling: I wanted the drug to wash away, dissolve into sleep, but it refused. My alarm clock—the kind whose numbers advanced one to the next like an old scoreboard—assumed a kind of malevolent force. It was so bright and the *clack* of each passing minute so loud, I had to cover it with a blanket. Our apartment building stood on a steep hill, and as cars struggled up the adjacent street, I could hear the gears groaning, engine pieces grinding together. Sparks could fly, I worried, and start a fire. I raced to the living room to watch out the window. From there, I was sure I could hear conversations from down the street. The sound of a bus chugging uphill made the walls vibrate.

I had no idea that other people also hallucinated while taking Halcion—and experienced worse side effects—until reports began to surface in the media in the early nineties. Halcion was reportedly linked to all sorts of psychotic mayhem. In his 1990 memoir *Darkness Visible*, novelist William Styron wrote how the drug exacerbated his clinical depression, leading him to become suicidal. The manufacturer of Halcion, Pharmacia & Upjohn, was slammed with dozens of lawsuits. The wife of a peaceful man who threw himself off a hotel roof while taking the drug won a $1.2-million settlement against the prescribing physician and an undisclosed amount from Upjohn. Banned in Great Britain in 1991, Halcion's been investigated time and again by the FDA since 1982, but never pulled from the American market. Instead, the drug was given a stricter warning label and its recommended dosage was changed.

Unaware of the controversy, I'd continued to use Halcion, sometimes two a night, at least once a week. Nick, who'd begun to have trouble sleeping himself, occasionally took half a pill, too. After about a year, the refills ran out. When I called to have the prescription renewed, the receptionist told me that Dr. Williamson had passed away. She didn't say how; she didn't have to. It was AIDS, I understood. The doctor who'd taken over his practice agreed to give me one more Halcion refill. But I knew I needed some other remedy. Nick and I moved to a new apartment; I thought I'd sleep better in a different place. We'd found a flat on a quiet street in a house with just one other tenant. But I'd unwittingly moved the problem with me. The incessant noise—the racket that really kept me awake—was in my head. By January of 1990, I was regularly leaving our bed to sleep on a futon in a walk-in closet under the stairs. Pitch-black, soundproof, it was like crawling inside an oven mitt. I may not always have slept soundly in there, but I fretted less about waking Nick.

I was always worrying about waking Nick—worrying, moreover, in daytime about what Nick would say or do about anything. It's possible that hypnotics altered my state of mind, yet I don't really think so. What I demanded of myself, and how I saw myself, caused enough damage. Although I had a good PR job at the San Francisco Museum of Modern Art, I felt unaccomplished. I didn't earn much money. I wanted to write; in what form and on what subject, however, I wasn't sure. Nick, an intense, competitive guy, made a good living; we drove a BMW and traveled a lot; he was generous. But our relationship had always centered on him. I was a satellite stuck in low orbit around his needs. I grew dissatisfied, frustrated. As did he, in some ways. Though we'd never pledged monogamy, by this stage we were both frequently out gratifying our individual libidinous whims. This reached its humiliating low point when, in a night of drunken confessions, Nick and I discovered that we'd both secretly had an affair at the same time with the same man, who, for his own amusement, I later learned, arranged some days to see us one right after the other.

The first time I ever woke up with Nick in his big cast-iron bed, I was surprised by something I hadn't noticed the night before: the sheets were pink. The finest Egyptian cotton in the most gorgeous coral-pink—chosen, he told me as we sipped freshly ground coffee in bed, because they made your skin and face look so rosy and youthful in the morning. After three and a half years together, I felt I'd become like those sheets: decorative, flattering to his appearance, and a little soiled, in need of changing. Friends were dead or dying of AIDS and here I was, healthy at age twenty-nine, letting my own life slip away.

I began to talk with him about separating but didn't act on it until one morning in early April 1990. A friend was heading to the airport for a week's vacation and suggested I stay at her place. It was the opening I needed. I stayed home from work, called Nick at his office, and told him I was leaving. I would take the bus and return later for my things. I packed a bag after doing a load of wash, folding our clothes, making the bed, and cleaning the kitchen. I left two Halcion tablets in the medicine cabinet for Nick and took the last three pills with me.

Chapter 15

≈

Fevers

TUESDAY, JULY 26, 1994. Afternoon: Here we are, in this car, at this moment, at this place we hoped never to be. I don't know which of us seems more lost and defeated. His seat belt buckled, Steve stares out the window. I think to myself wearily, we haven't even gotten home yet and we've already moved to a new place. We are itinerants, our old lives wiped out, the future stretching no more than a few miles. He is planning for the next stop. I am in charge of driving.

I cannot help retracing our steps, frantically searching for something of intense personal value, lost within the space of a few minutes, a few city blocks. We had walked from the parking garage, through the heavy office doors, and into the waiting room, where we took our seats. We've done it so often, we could have found it in our sleep. A nurse brought us into a tiny, overheated room. I sat in a chair, Steve on the exam table, and we waited anxiously, as though stuck in a broken-down elevator, for the door to open.

His doctor, Marge, appeared and began casually leafing through Steve's file, as if she were looking for a telephone number. He peeked over her shoulder. "So, am I in the land of AIDS?" He said it playfully, covering for fear, as if he were guessing at a riddle.

With a childlike sense of denial that seemed rational at the time, I furiously prayed to one of my dead friends to stop time and magically switch around the T-cell numbers. My daydream was interrupted by Marge. She was speaking very, very slowly. "You are . . . in the land . . . of AIDS. . . ."

The next thing I remember, we were back on the sidewalk. I felt just as I did off the fourteen-hour flight to Berlin for the International AIDS Conference the summer before: exhausted, grimy, disoriented. Looking for signs in English—and finding none. I couldn't think of anything to say other than, "I'll get the car." Steve leaned against the building and I ran to the parking garage.

Pulling up to the curb, I flashed on the first time I'd seen Steve: morning, December 26, 1989, at Muscle System, a gym on Hayes Street. I was knocked out by his beautiful physique; flattop, shaved chest; sweet grin, handsome face. Plugged into a Walkman, he danced between sets. "Oh, boy, this one's trouble," I said to myself; I was still living with Nick. And then I heard Steve's accent when we flirted near the locker room: native New Jersey, no question about it—one of my favorite sounds. He was like a late Christmas present: a total surprise. Michelangelo's *David* in a baggy pair of gym shorts.

Steve was twenty-six, three years younger than me. He'd moved to San Francisco from Chicago a couple of years before. Though we were clearly attracted to each other, Steve wasn't keen on getting involved with "a married man." He kept a safe distance until Nick and I broke up. Which is not to say we didn't secretly see each other in the interim. He visited me at the art museum, I'd drop by the restaurant where he worked as a waiter. Over dinner one night early on, he told me that he was HIV-positive.

I wasn't completely shocked. Most men I knew either had AIDS or hadn't yet taken the test, being both too fearful to learn the results and realistic enough to understand there was little one could do anyway until he got sick. (Just one AIDS-defining "opportunistic infection," *Pneumocystis carinii* pneumonia [PCP], was treatable, even preventable.) Hence, the operating assumption when dating was that everyone was HIV-infected—even if they said they were HIV-negative. Still, I was surprised by Steve's disclosure. He didn't have "that look" at all; indeed, at six foot one, 190 pounds, he was unusually fit and muscular.

A waiter had broken in to clear away plates, putting our conversation on pause. I then neglected to disclose my own status when Steve and I resumed talking. I had no idea this had left him out on a limb, dangling, for the rest of the meal. On some level, I think I felt guilty: I'd been lucky. Steve seemed calm, poised, yet later said he'd felt nervous about how I'd react: "Telling people your status is like riding a roller coaster—you can do it a hundred times but each time it still makes you a little sick." As we walked back to his apartment from the restaurant, he bluntly asked my status and I told him.

Steve's revelation didn't scare me away; it drew me in. Attracted to his strength and candor and romantic idealism—

perhaps hoping some would rub off—I walked over to see him late in the afternoon on the day I left Nick. I gave Steve my news, then he announced his: He'd just seen his doctor, who'd given him his "numbers," the results from blood tests that quantify the virus's activity and the immune system's strength. Steve's T cells were down, nothing alarming yet not a good sign. There was a new theory that treating HIV infection before symptoms appeared might keep serious illnesses at bay, so he'd been given a prescription for AZT. Steve took his first two capsules right then—on an empty stomach, purposely, so he could feel it in his body. We celebrated by going out to buy a year's supply of condoms and a pillow for when I'd spend the night.

In July, I gave up the apartment I'd rented for myself and moved into Steve's studio. I had more stuff than when I'd first moved to San Francisco, but not much. Still, it barely fit into the few empty spaces left in Steve's small, dark apartment on Bush near Fillmore. The last item was my bed, the futon from the closet under the stairs. There was nowhere left to put it, so I stacked it on top of his.

It worried my friends and family that I'd moved in with Steve just four months after breaking up with Nick—as well as that he was HIV-positive, of course. "Yeah, it's all happening very quickly," I'd reassure them, "but what can I say? I want a future with him." The obsessive clock-watching of an insomniac was gradually transformed; I began to take a longer view of how well I was spending my hours awake. Given all that Steve was doing to stay healthy, recreational drug use and drinking no longer appealed. I stopped taking Halcion. My first magazine article was published that summer—a freelance reporting piece for *Mother Jones* on young gay men and attitudes about AIDS—after which I turned more seriously to writing, attempting to shape material from turgid journal entries into personal essays.

My sleep patterns changed. As a waiter, Steve worked

late and went to bed late, two or three in the morning; he was a great companion when I couldn't sleep. We'd talk in the kitchen for hours; watch *Star Trek* reruns on TV; go shopping at midnight at Safeway. Some nights, we'd go out dancing. Once home, we'd peel off our sweat-drenched T-shirts and jeans, have sex, take a shower together. I didn't think quite so much about sleeping. Which is not to say I wasn't often tired. I had to be up by seven to commute to a new job at the modern art museum in Berkeley.

Since I was already up, I'd wake Steve every morning so he could take his pills. Instead of his getting out of bed, I brought the pills to him—two white capsules of AZT and one blue capsule of Acyclovir, each imprinted with a tiny black unicorn and the company name Wellcome, a rather ironic greeting. I can see myself, dressed for work, kneeling on the futons, hesitating a moment before putting my hand on his bare arm. I'd never liked waking anyone. "Hey, bub," I whisper affectionately. He doesn't move. Then, louder, and with a shake: "Hey. You."

"Hey." He sits up. Dazed by the sunlight and without his glasses, Steve's green eyes wander slightly, giving his pillow-wrinkled face the look of a felled boxer, seeing stars, leaning against the ropes. I drop the capsules in one of his palms, push a glass of water into the other. "For me?" he cracks, then swallows the pills and falls back asleep for three hours, when he'll get up for another round.

❧

At ten capsules a day, AZT made a powerful impact, though not solely on the virus. Steve woke late every morning with a head-dulling "AZT buzz" and often felt nauseous. He said he could smell AZT in his pee, on his skin. Before long, other drugs and supplements were added to Steve's daily schedule.

Three mornings a week, I gave him an injection in his shoulder of an experimental immune-system booster called Iscador. A supply would arrive by Express Mail from Switzerland where it was manufactured—twenty-four ampoules neatly wrapped and boxed, like expensive chocolates. Iscador was an extract made from mistletoe—a lovely idea, I thought, with its hint of a Christmas kiss. And, it turned out, just as innocuous.

Steve remained in good health overall, free of symptoms ("asymptomatic"), and continued to work full-time as a waiter. We saved enough money to move in the spring of 1991 and found a one-bedroom on the edge of Pacific Heights. After our application had been approved, I met with the building manager, Jorge, to pick up the keys. Steve was working, so I'd gone on my own.

Jorge, a Latino man in his late thirties, walked me through the freshly painted apartment for a routine inspection. He said he'd lived in the building for ten years. "The people downstairs can be a little noisy, I'm told, and the wall heaters don't crank out much heat," he confided, "but the light's great. And not a bad view." Through the large bedroom windows, he pointed out Twin Peaks in the distance and a sliver of Lafayette Park up beyond California Street.

I told him how much Steve and I loved the apartment.

"It's nice to have another gay couple here," he said.

"Oh, you have a better half?"

"Well, Keith." After a pause, Jorge said quietly, "He died last year."

AIDS, I thought, before Jorge said it himself, as though I already knew. "I'm so sorry."

Standing in the empty bedroom with its blank, white walls, I automatically thought of our friends Rob and Peter, a couple who'd lived on the opposite edge of our new neighborhood. Both had recently died of AIDS, one right after the other. The certainty of their togetherness was evidenced by a

wild, painted mural they'd begun years earlier in their bedroom. An extension of their matching panther tattoos, the
elaborate mural was a tropical jungle of lush life—huge
fronds, exotic birds, half-hidden predators. Beautiful, bright,
and never finished. The idea of doing something so permanent
to these white walls was perpendicular to Steve's and my parallel thoughts. We felt guilty drilling the first hole, hanging the
first picture. We'd bought Spackle at the same time as screws.

The possibility of Steve following Rob and Peter and
Keith had given our relationship an intense clarity. In the beginning, I'd considered Steve "my lover"—that's how I introduced and referred to him, as he did me. But in our first year
together, a revision had taken place. Without ceremony, we'd
become partners. He helped me with my writing—reading
and editing every draft of my work, and every proposal letter.
Saturdays were art-review days. I'd gotten my first regular freelance gig writing reviews of photography shows for *Art Week*.
Any pretensions I might've had were punctured by Steve, a
voice of mercilessness and humor in the antiseptic galleries.
Of course, he was no less honest when it came time to review
what I had written. Though I received just $30 per piece, I'd
rework numerous drafts he'd marked up until every word
counted.

I served a similar role for Steve. Together, we'd found
him a whip-smart new doctor, a wonderfully direct, acerbic
woman named Marge Poscher, and I joined Steve at every appointment. We researched the latest drugs. We attended Project Inform's community meetings on clinical trials and new
treatments. In September of that year, I stood in line at an underground Buyer's Club to buy Steve two bottles of the antiviral drug ddC. In preliminary trials, ddC had been the first
drug since AZT to offer any promise of slowing the virus. We
had waited two months for the drug to come in. I got a six-
month supply, the most they'd sell me, for $120 cash.

"Do you want a bag?" the clerk had asked.

"Yes, please." I left feeling that I had in my possession something illegal. As a matter of fact, I did: ddC had not yet been approved by the FDA. I carried the bag directly over to the Mexican restaurant where Steve was then working and stopped him on his way to the kitchen.

"I got it."

Holding it from view under a bar table, I opened the bottle and pulled out the cotton ball. We peered inside at four hundred icy-white capsules. "That's it?" Steve asked. "Is that all there is?" Each capsule was tiny, just a few milligrams of chemicals blown into a gelatin egg. How could we know if it was the right powder, the right drug? Was there enough ddC in each capsule or too much? This stash was cooked up in someone's basement, we knew, not dispensed at our neighborhood pharmacy.

One slippery capsule jumped from the bottle and bounced onto the tile floor. It was so small, Steve couldn't pick it up with his large, heavy fingers. At that moment, it crossed my mind: This is a prop. The drug, in its white bottle with the generic label, is a fake, nothing more.

I wet my fingers, reached down to pick up the capsule, and dropped it into Steve's palm. He swallowed the ddC and gave me a kiss. "Cheers," I said.

"Let's hope it works," he said.

"Yes, let's."

And we did. We *hoped* longer than was perhaps sensible, given ddC's unpleasant side effects—nausea, cramping—and several months longer than the drug probably worked. But we were driven and, for the first time, a little scared. There were no other options and Steve's T cells had started to thin out. One night I had a dream that we were knocking at my friend Ken's door. He answered.

"Hi," I said tentatively, unsure what tone to strike. "So, we heard that you are well. That you don't have it anymore."

"Yeah," he replied calmly. "Now I'm just trying to live without it." We all laughed nervously.

"Well, what did you do?" Steve asked. "What did you take? Who's your doctor?"

Ken started to answer, but someone called to him from within the house. "Sorry, I'll be back in a minute," he promised. "Wait here."

Steve and I waited and waited at the door. But Ken never returned to tell us how he had been cured.

Our waking life took on the quality of that unresolved dream: we stood together, supported each other, *sure* that the answer would come, but skeptical, too, tired of waiting.

In late 1991, I started a job at the San Francisco AIDS Foundation. As a member of the education department, I was responsible for creating media campaigns promoting "early treatment for HIV," precisely the kind of regimen Steve followed. With his positive attitude and tremendous self-discipline, he was my inspiration for a national series of billboards, ads, and public-service announcements, plus T-shirts, buttons, and other free items, with the hopeful tag line "Be Here for the Cure." Steve began working at the AIDS Foundation himself, first as a hot-line volunteer and then, in the summer of 1993, as a full-time staff person. Now thirty years old, Steve was a trained peer counselor for gay men, many of them HIV-positive —a job he loved.

Around that time, Steve began to exhibit early physical symptoms of HIV disease: fungal infections, low-grade fevers, and stretches of fatigue. It was not unusual for him to sleep twelve hours per night and take naps on weekends. Marge said this was to be expected: his medications were powerful; the stress of having a chronic illness takes a toll; and he was fighting off infections. I later learned, too, that the sleep of people with HIV is damaged just like their immune systems. As the disease progresses, it disrupts basic physiological systems, such as body temperature rhythms and the timing of hormone secretions; as a result, the structure of sleep changes. A period of deep, non-REM sleep, for example, may arrive out of sequence at the very end of the night (rather than in the first third). In general, people with HIV take longer to fall asleep, get less deep sleep, and awaken more frequently, all of which leaves them drowsier in daytime.

While fatigue and sleep disturbances reflect a decline in health, there's no doubt that sleep is healing. Researchers say that deep, non-REM sleep serves, in part, as a time for the body to repair and the immune system to strengthen. Growth hormone, for instance, which is essential for tissue repair and in mediating the sleep-promoting activity of infection-fighting cytokines, is secreted by the pineal gland in one or two large pulses only during sleep stages 3 and 4.

It was possible then for me to view my old nemesis, sleep, as an ally for Steve. But not always. Some nights he woke two or three times with night sweats. Sound asleep, he had no awareness of their coming, no chance to fend them off. Steve said it was as shocking as someone sneaking up in the dark and dousing him with a bucket of water. After each episode, he was soaking wet—not just his T-shirt and underwear, but sheets, pillow, mattress cover, as if his body had flushed everything out at once. Come morning, it looked as if a snowman had perished on his side of the bed. The sweats tended to come in clusters—three or four nights consecutively, then none for several weeks. Their unpredictability was

unsettling. I remember waking with him and the split second
of panic as I felt his cold, wet skin. We sprang into action: he
toweled off, I grabbed clean sheets. On such nights, I thought
it took guts for him to go back to sleep at all.

The next day, the clammy sheets and clothes balled up in
the laundry closet smelled sour, an odor of sickness that was
new to our home. It washed out. Yet after I took bedsheets
from the dryer, folded and put them away, questions still hung
in the air. Why was Steve's body responding so brutally? Were
night sweats a good sign, a fever breaking, or a bad one, complete immune-system breakdown? As Steve once put it, bewil-
dered after the third drenching in a single night, "How many
times can a fever break?"

Doctors still cannot explain their torrential nature.
Though related to body temperature regulation, the exact
cause and purpose of night sweats is not known. Biologists say
that breaking into a cold sweat can be a natural response to
fear, with the heart racing and blood pumping into the legs. I
imagine that when Steve started having night sweats, his
body—trapped in a fever loop—was also reacting to the danger it faced, as though in a dream it had glimpsed the future.

A few times, I woke to Steve having nightmares. He
kicked his legs and cried out. I pushed my legs to his, to muf-
fle the blows, and put my hand to his chest. He turned over
and quieted. In one dream, Steve later told me, his strong,
white teeth turned rotten. He spit them out, mouthful after
mouthful, like bloody gravel. In another, he was trying to lick a
postage stamp, of all things, but had no saliva left to moisten
it. Weakened by HIV in real life, Steve's body failed him in
dreams, part by part.

His worst recurring nightmare was that he was blinded
by CMV retinitis, his eyesight lost to insoluble black spots. In
the dream, his attempts at learning braille were useless: nerve

damage had destroyed the sense of touch in his hands. This would be his body's ultimate betrayal, Steve told me: he could no longer see, read, feel.

Steve started on ddI after ddC failed. He also began exploring "alternative" therapies. From one of his clients, he'd heard about DNCB, which was sold at the Buyer's Club. DNCB (dinitrochlorobenzene) was originally created as a chemical for developing photographs; it had been reinvented by "anti-antiviral" AIDS activists as a treatment for HIV disease. One evening Steve came home with four small brown-glass bottles, bundled together with a rubber band along with a set of instructions—a "DNCB kit" purchased for $25. Ironically, the bottles looked exactly like poppers—vials of amyl nitrite, an inhalant used to enhance orgasms.

Following the highly detailed, typed instructions, I used a cotton swab to paint a two-by-two-inch square of strong-smelling, yellowish liquid on Steve's inner biceps. The theory was that the immune system would be shocked into action by poisoning the skin and, therefore, mount a renewed attack on HIV infection. For good measure, I repainted the square, then covered it with a bandage. In hours, it caused a chemical burn so painful—"like acid burning through my skin and muscles, down to my bone," Steve later said—that he couldn't sleep. At 2 A.M., in excruciating pain, he tried to wash it from his blistered skin. Steve finally fell asleep at dawn, holding a bag of ice to his arm.

Exactly as the instructions prescribed, Steve did a second DNCB treatment two weeks later (from the second, stronger of the four bottles) on the opposite arm. The pain was intense, he noted, but he didn't complain. He had a phenomenal ability to separate himself from physical discomfort, to focus on the smallest gleam of consciousness that wasn't enflamed and sink into it, as if in a sensory-deprivation chamber. Which meant zoning me out as well. The depth of his perseverance was way beyond my understanding. He continued to use DNCB regularly, along with ddI, AZT, and the other drugs. By January of 1994, Steve's inner arms bore square, rust-colored DNCB scars—like tattoos—marks that were recognizable to other DNCB users in the "AIDS community." I developed a strange body marking of my own: a bald patch on the back of my head, the size of a silver dollar. Some people thought it was a hip-hop haircut. At one of Steve's appointments, Marge glanced at it and instantly diagnosed it as alopecia, a symptom of acute anxiety. When I asked her what she'd prescribe, she said, "A vacation."

As for Steve, she told him to begin taking yet a fourth antiviral drug, d4T, because his T cells were plummeting, he'd started to have diarrhea, and he'd lost weight. I began to suspect that DNCB might be to blame. The stress caused by pain and discomfort was immune-*suppressing*, I hypothesized, rather than immune-boosting. I was desperate to blame his deteriorating health on something within our control—something other than HIV. One Sunday afternoon, as he pulled the DNCB bottle from the refrigerator, I told Steve my theory. "Plus," I added, "my concerns are self-centered. On DNCB days, you're so out of it that I'm robbed of a whole day with you." He was silent when I finished my rehearsed speech. "So," I said, "what do you think? Are you going to keep using it?"

"Yes, absolutely."

I was furious. "Steve, did you even hear me? If you're going to conduct an experiment on your body, there's got to be some clinical proof that it's working."

"Okay," he spit back, "well, you just tell me what clinical markers would satisfy you."

His sarcasm stopped me. "Look, the point is," I said, rattled, "the point is . . ." I'd lost my point. "I want to be sure it's doing what you want it to do."

"God, you just don't get it, do you? What I want it to do

is to save my life!" he yelled. "I want it to save my life. I don't
know if I can ever give you sufficient proof of that."

⤛

As I felt the epidemic overtake my life, I fought off insomnia
as one fights to stave off sleep, but its pull was overwhelming.
I saw AIDS at work, at the gym, at home. And when I didn't
see it in other people's lives, my resentment seethed. This was
the summer of 1994, a period that can be captured in a single
scene.

It is nighttime. I am sitting in bed reading and trying not
to notice the downstairs neighbor's laughter. Rather, I am trying not to be irritated by it. The laughter has a far greater presence than the neighbor himself. He has lived there three years
and I have never seen him in the flesh. I cannot imagine his
looks. I can barely hear his voice—can't make out any
words—through our floor, his ceiling. But I know him by the
sound of his laughter. Four big, juicy notes: *ha-ha, ha-ha.*

I can't stand it anymore. I point my finger at the floor,
like a pistol, and say I want to kill him. The neighbor could
save himself easily, I allow, if he would just stop laughing.
Steve remains safely undercover, absorbed in a science-fiction
paperback. I pull the finger-trigger. "Bang!"

Ha-ha, ha-ha.

"Missed," Steve says without glancing up from his book.

It wasn't just noise, you see—any more than, say, cockroaches in a kitchen are just pests. The laughter lived here,
along with the middle-of-the-night car alarms and predawn
garbage trucks, the upstairs dog's tail-thumping and the next-
door neighbor's country music, and Steve and HIV and me.
Each had its effect on the other. Each had its role to play. In
the laughter I heard the hallucinatory sound of a person living

his life carelessly—literally without cares—and taunting my partner and me. I would've done anything to protect us from it.

The laughter got louder when the sun went down. It left during the day, returned to hunt at night. It fairly screamed up to us: I am young; I am healthy; I have a full life in front of me. Some nights, I hardly noticed it. Others, it was like a pack howling from under our bed. Steve, ill from a severe allergic reaction to a new drug, put his book down one night and murmured that he was sick and tired of being sick and tired, and the laughter filled in the silence where I didn't know what to say.

It was so much harder than he could ever have imagined, Steve admitted. He wondered what it would have been like if he had never tested for HIV. If he had lived in blissful ignorance until one day, without warning, he up and died. The laughter waited silently at the foot of our bed. Steve didn't even notice it, as if his defenses were tuned to a different frequency.

He asked how the infection on his feet looked, and as I examined it, the laughter shot through the floorboards. He mentioned that, with his doctor's appointment this coming Friday, he could receive an AIDS diagnosis if his T cells had dropped below two hundred. He said that it was time to add my name to his bank account, to obtain a living will. He asked if I could handle it if he got really sick.

Yes, of course, I answered. I didn't mention that I was terrified.

The laughter exploded.

Steve would remind me that it was a lot better than the previous neighbors—"the cokeheads," I contemptuously called them—who sometimes kept us up half the night bingeing, laughing, screaming at each other, then noisily having sex, and finally, snoring. But I kind of missed them. I felt better than them. They always looked tweaked-out and disheveled as I rushed by them, the morning after, on my way to work. Our current neighbor, an imaginary paradigm of modern normalcy, was more disturbing. Like an alien from another planet, he spoke a different, wordless language, consisting of only two distinct sounds: the laughter and the moan. Sometimes the moan made *me* laugh. We'd hear it twice a week, always on Sunday nights at about 11 P.M. and then sometime midweek.

It was the inverse of the laugh, except there were three notes, not four, and they were delivered more slowly: *ah-ah-ah, ah-ah-ah*. His female partner provided the soprano harmony. The moan was time-limited, too, lasting about twenty minutes. Unlike the laughter, I always knew it would end.

It sounded like bad, vanilla pornography. "Ah-ah-ah!" I mimicked during an especially loud session, rolling on top of Steve and gleefully contorting my face. He pushed me off and made me promise to shut up. I made fun of it, but the moan got under my skin as much as the laughter. It was the sound of people living their lives without fear, without rules. It said: We are straight; we are uninfected; we don't have safe sex— we don't have to. It mocked the two of us upstairs, sitting in bed quietly reading night after night, week after week, without having sex (because he didn't feel well or I was depressed), or lying side by side mutually masturbating.

We kissed good-night and turned off the lights. I wondered what the laugher heard from below. Just footsteps, I imagined, as if an Etch A Sketch traced our nightly course on the downstairs ceiling. Steve was out of bed twice before falling asleep at twelve. We woke up at one-thirty when the night sweats, like a warm island downpour—here and gone in a heartbeat—drenched the bed. I stayed up till three in the company of a Fred Flintstone jelly glass filled with wine, then lay awake in bed for another two hours. Following my seven o'clock alarm, I returned with a handful of Steve's pills, the day's first dose.

The fury of nighttime was gone, replaced by a frazzled exhaustion. The laughter was silent. I sat on the edge of the bed and watched Steve sleep. Four and a half years of this wake-up ritual and it still seemed slightly cruel, almost unethical. I wished he could sleep dreamlessly for days; it seemed like the healthiest immunotherapy for him. Although his breathing was silent, the bedcovers rose and fell in soft waves. Arms braided, he clutched a pillow under his turned head. I couldn't see his face. And I suddenly felt a mixture of fear and sadness that left me even more exhausted. I understood what sleep scientists meant when they said, paradoxically, you can live without sleep, yet sleep is necessary for survival. At that moment, I was so tired I didn't know how I was going to make it.

Tuesday, July 26, 1994. Evening: Here we are, in the last aisle, at the end of the row, at this place we do not really wish to be. We had bought circus tickets weeks before. Exhausted and uninterested, we had nevertheless been unable to think of a good reason not to use them. Huddled together for warmth, we hold hands beneath our crossed legs. Ushers close the heavy canvas door-flaps. Lights go out, music comes up, a spotlight snaps on. The show begins.

A corps of acrobats emerges from the darkness dressed in sparkling green leotards and head caps. Like caterpillars nibbling at a leaf, they gently pull away pieces of the green flooring. Trampolines are stretched seamlessly underneath. The acrobats line up, sprint, and the moment they hit the trampolines, fly into space.

One after another, they gracefully throw their bodies into

the air and are transformed into birds, twisting, spinning, defying gravity as they climb higher and higher. Sometimes their leaps are so high, they have ages to dive in a thrilling, slow-motion free fall. It seems as if I have a lifetime to watch. But each finishes in a flash, replaced in midair by another. As the act reaches its climax, two acrobats vault at once from opposite sides, their bodies dangerously—and flawlessly—interweaving.

I watch the acrobats flying. It is so beautiful—painfully beautiful, like looking into the sun—I have to shut my eyes. In their elegant leaps into space and falls to earth, time is infinite. I can see everything, ineffably, at once.

I turn to Steve, perched uncomfortably on the hard wooden bench: his future clipped, his exquisite body falling. And his life strikes me not simply as tragic, but—like the acrobat's leap—as sublime, breathtaking: speeded up, a series of complex twists and turns, of beauty and pain, courage and fear, skill and daring, over in a moment. I realize I cannot save Steve. Nor can I only watch. But I can throw my body into midair with his.

෴

Chapter 16

Fatal Familial Insomnia

What keeps human beings tense and sometimes
wakeful is a fact independent of epoch or era.
That is man's ability to project into the future.
It is doubtful, for example, that any other
animal knows it is going to die.

—Nathaniel Kleitman

STEVE OFTEN said I'd make a terrible sick person—as in, a terminally ill person. He wasn't being disparaging so much as frank. I deeply resented this charge—preferring to view myself as a model of stoicism—but he was right, I had to admit. "Well, *you'd* make a terrible caregiver!" I'd shoot back. That always got a laugh. I contended that the very qualities that made me unsuited to being sick made me well suited to caregiving: pity, a genius for worrying, the ability to exaggerate symptoms. Getting a cold or flu, for example, made me panicky. I wanted to be well in an instant. In part, I was afraid of making Steve sick. In part, I was mildly hypochondriacal, just like my father. But I also felt responsible for keeping my life orderly as an antidote to the turbulence in Steve's. In October of 1994, I'd started a demanding full-time job in fund-raising for San Francisco's Main Library and continued to write in my spare time while also taking care of the household chores. So if my physical energy evaporated, I flipped out. Nothing made me more irrational than insomnia.

One night in a six-night bout remains vivid. I lay awake next to Steve and thought, I would steal an hour of his sleep if I could. I would slip beneath his eyelids and yank it right out of him. He would feel nothing. Nor would I—neither remorse nor shame. One hour of perfect unconsciousness: one clean, soundless dive, deeper and deeper, as far as my lungs would take me. I would come up for air before he woke.

Instead, I lay motionless, as though sewn to the sheets by the smallest demons, watching Steve's silhouette against the bedroom blinds. Fondness became hostility: How does he do this for eight hours? I listened to his tranquil breathing, furious that he slept while I could not. Finally, at 3 A.M., I snipped the threads, discarded my carcass at bedside, and left it behind in disgust. Time for the insomniac to make his rounds.

I crept into the next room, where I felt a thrilling freedom from my own body. I was naked, but not cold; not thirsty or hungry; I could smell nothing. My eyesight was shot; I couldn't face the TV, work, or read. The plug had been kicked out of the socket, the circadian clock stopped, and I roamed the apartment of my own power, on my own theory of time, occupying a fragile space between dreaming and functioning.

It would not last beyond daylight, I knew. As always, the panic swooped in around 5 A.M. and I found myself on the couch, burrowing under a blanket, shivering. Light began to filter in. I covered my head with my arms, convinced that the darker I made it, the more likely I would sleep. But I did not sleep.

Every so often, Steve begged to differ with my morning-after reports. Adamant that I hadn't slept more than an hour the night before, for instance, I'd be shocked to hear him say, "You were sound asleep from three to five, at least. I was in and out of the bathroom twice and awake myself."

"No way, I just had my eyes closed."

"You were snoring."

Uh-oh, caught in a lie that I didn't even know I'd committed. Isn't that a sign of schizophrenia? In point of fact, insomniacs are notoriously bad judges of the amount we sleep. This has been proved in sleep laboratories, where a person's memory of, say, three lousy hours' sleep is clearly contradicted next morning by an EEG indicating a solid six. This is not so much a bid for sympathy from doctors and good sleepers, I believe, as it is a symptom of a mind so exhausted it's on the blink. Like an anorexic who prefers the sight of bones sticking through skin, a chronic insomniac may take a twisted pride in his or her sleeplessness. In an extreme form, this may indicate a psychological disorder called sleep state misperception, in which, all evidence to the contrary, a person claims to be an incurable insomniac.

"A bit of personal experience may serve to emphasize this important fact," Dr. H. M. Johnson observed in 1928. He was a guest at a summer cottage along with a woman who was "badly run down from long subjection to an unavoidable and exacting domestic problem. She suffered, as she believed, also from insomnia." She went to bed early and slept poorly, she told Dr. Johnson and the other guests over breakfast, meticulously accounting for her wakefulness at every hour.

Dr. Johnson himself lay awake one night. "As the house was by no means soundproof, I was able to assure the lady the next day that she was getting more sleep than she supposed; for during a considerable part of the time she had credited to wakefulness she had been making respiratory noises such as no lady of her birth and breeding would have made if she had known what she was doing."

The lady rejected the doctor's breakfast testimony, exactly as I would Steve's. It made me angry when he disagreed, telling me I'd slept; telling me I didn't look tired at all; no, I didn't have bags under my eyes. I had become an unreliable narrator in a story in which my situation—indeed, my character—was other than that which I claimed. I not only overstated the amount of sleep I lost, but its effect on me. Sometimes I felt as if I hadn't slept well in weeks and that I never would again. I became secretly convinced that my pounding headaches were symptoms of a brain tumor and, most disturbingly, that I had sero-converted. There was no rational reason to think I'd become HIV-positive—and an HIV test later showed I hadn't—but I couldn't think of another explanation for my frequent colds and low-grade fevers.

Lying awake, I didn't try to recollect my life, as I had since I was a boy. I spun macabre stories about the future. I was sure Steve was going to die suddenly: I would either wake up to find him dead next to me or come home to find his cold, lifeless body in bed. I played out different scenarios of what I should do: call his doctor Marge, call 911, call my friends Steven and Garth. No, no, no: first call Steven and Garth, then 911, then call Marge. Where would I hold the memorial? What music would he want played? Oh, and a reminder to myself: before you pronounce him dead, check first to make sure he's not breathing! And for God's sake, take a CPR class at the Red Cross.

As one might imagine, none of this was sleep-inducing. The sicker Steve got, the more difficulty I had with sleep—an equation so simple as to seem scarcely worth mentioning. In the thick of it, though, I had little perspective of what was wrong with me. I interpreted my insomnia as a physical and moral failure; in retrospect, I see it differently. If sleep is a kind of death, as people have often said, then insomnia is a sign of life—"the horror of being and going on being," as Jorge Luis Borges wrote in his 1981 poem "Two Forms of Insomnia." It is *longevity*, consciousness of a lifetime, expressed in a single night: ". . . being well aware that I am bound to my flesh, to a voice I detest, to my name, to routinely remembering. . . . It is trying to sink into death and being unable to sink into death. It is being and continuing to be."

Of course, one can choose either to fight it or go with it. Or, as I did occasionally, to dodge it: I started taking sleeping pills again for the first time in five years. That is, what I assumed to be sleeping pills: my doctor prescribed Xanax, an antianxiety medication. I remember standing in the bathroom at 1 A.M., sticking my tongue out, and watching myself place a Xanax on it: "I am taking a sleeping pill," I would say, to impress it upon my brain and prevent myself from inadvertently taking more than one. "I am going to sleep," and yet often I wouldn't.

Had I known about it at the time, I'd surely have feared I was suffering from "fatal familial insomnia." This rare brain-wasting disease begins with severe insomnia, followed by bizarre phobias and hallucinations, and always ends in death. Fatal familial insomnia (FFI) literally destroys the mind. It was first identified in 1985, the same year the related "mad cow disease" was first observed in British cattle. Both are "prion diseases," caused by defective cellular proteins known as prions. Different prion diseases attack different parts of the brain. FFI damages the thalamus. A small, egg-shaped structure at the core of the brain, near the hypothalamus, the thalamus normally serves as a relay station for messages from the sense organs to specific sensory areas of the cerebral cortex.

In FFI, it is hypothesized, the mechanisms that block sensory input gradually fail, so the body is never able to shut out alerting impulses and "cross over" from wakefulness. Falling asleep becomes a physiological impossibility.

Since it was first described by Dr. Elio Lugaresi and colleagues at the University of Bologna, no treatments for FFI have been found. The frightful course of disease, however, has been thoroughly documented. In the early eighties a fifty-three-year-old Italian man found himself suddenly unable to nap during the day, as had been his custom, or to sleep more than three hours per night. An industrial manager who had previously seen his father and two sisters die following similar early symptoms, this man became Dr. Lugaresi's first FFI patient. Three months after onset, the insomnia had become almost total and was now associated with brief, vivid dreamlike episodes, which the man acted out in a fashion similar to people with REM behavior disorder. Bodily functions rapidly disintegrated; within five months of his first symptoms, this formerly healthy man was in a continuous stupor. In the end stage, his circadian rhythms malfunctioned; melatonin secretion, for instance, no longer elevated at nighttime. When FFI Case #1 died, he'd gone without normal sleep for at least six months.

Background investigations by Dr. Lugaresi and colleagues revealed that FFI had likely affected twenty-eight members of this one Italian family over six generations. Autopsies confirmed seven cases. Five other unrelated families with FFI have reportedly been identified: another in Italy, one in Bordeaux, France, and three in the United States. FFI strikes between ages thirty and sixty and progresses to death as early as seven months after the first symptoms. DNA studies have pinpointed the inherited genetic error that triggers it: a mutation at codon 178 of the prion protein gene located on chromosome 20, which sounds more like an intergalactic address than a bodily one. In 1999, scientists at the University of California, San Francisco, identified a second form of fatal insomnia, similar in all respects to FFI except for one: it is not hereditary but occurs spontaneously. In other words, "sporadic fatal insomnia," as it's been called, could theoretically happen to anyone.

Prior to the extensive research on FFI, the role of the thalamus in regulating sleep was relatively unexplored. The study of FFI is considered equally important for a second reason. This horrible disease appears to prove what scientists of the past could only speculate and what chronic insomniacs had long imagined: if sleep disappears completely, death occurs.

While total-sleep-deprivation experiments have been done repeatedly with lab rats and dogs, the longest verified period a human subject had been kept awake was for just over a week. In 1957, at age sixty-two, Nathaniel Kleitman himself went without sleep for seven and a half days—180 hours. His eyes burned unbearably, he saw double, and the desire for sleep was almost unconquerable, but he did not get seriously ill, and there were no striking changes in his vital signs. Instead, he later reported, his judgment and self-control diminished, indicating "a fatigue of the higher levels of the cerebral cortex." Dr. Kleitman was only able to stay awake by using amphetamines. As he noted, though, in ordinary situations one need not resort to stimulants: "Worry is an excellent preventive of sleep," he said at the time. "Our peculiar gift of looking forward lets us worry about all probable misfortunes and many improbable ones."

～～

I took to sitting at the window in our living room when I had insomnia. With my Walkman on, I could distract my mind from its grimmest imaginings. There I am on a typical night: lights out, I pull the blinds up and settle in to watch the neighborhood from our couch. Spying on all the activity, both routine and random, makes me feel calm and superior. I like the streetlight on Pine, blinking red in the middle of the night. It keeps time with the music: Joni Mitchell, *Turbulent Indigo*. The Middle Eastern homeless man shows up, pushing his grocery cart up Octavia, crossing Pine, his regular route. I pull off my headphones and hear the percussive rattle of the hundred crushed cans in his cart. He parks it in front of the Catholic church and, for no discernible reason, yells wildly in Arabic before falling to his knees in supplication, kissing the sidewalk, bowing many times, then standing to face north, east, south, and west and say an incoherent prayer aloud. "You crazy fuck," I murmur affectionately. He sleeps in the church's gardens, at the feet of a statue of the Virgin Mary.

Up the street, the intersection at Octavia and California is dangerous, the only one in this area without a streetlight. Collisions are common. I can see them happening in advance, as if I'm watching a slow-motion film in driver's ed. That Jeep there—the one that hardly paused at Pine—it's going too fast up Octavia, it's going to roll through the stop sign at California. With the blind spot caused by all the parked cars, the driver's not going to see if a car's racing down California—*bang!* Sure enough, the Jeep clips the Lexus as it swerves into the left lane. No one's hurt, which is good. I can see the two drivers get out of their cars and argue, gesturing broadly as if pantomiming for a distant audience.

I loved telling Steve these stories the next day—stories of other people's misfortunes. One drama, however, I kept to myself—that of the gay couple in the building midway up the block. In their lives I took vicarious pleasure. No older than us, they lived in a swanky, first-floor apartment with a large back patio and solarium clearly visible from our place. Some weekend nights, they threw parties. By 2 A.M., when I assumed my perch, the festivities might be in full swing, men and women dancing, alcohol obviously loosening up things. During just such a soiree, I saw one member of the gay couple sneak through the solarium and out onto the patio with another man. Their faces visible under a patio light, they crept to the far dark corner and started necking, one man's hand up the other's shirt. Then, the other partner appeared at the solarium door. It was like a scene out of a farce. I wanted to open my window and holler, "No, don't go out there! Not a step farther!" And to the philandering one, "Stop! Pull yourself together!" They must have telepathically picked up my messages, for the good partner retreated back into the apartment, without seeing a thing, and the bad one stepped away from his drunken crush and walked indoors.

The good one knew I watched. I turned on a light one night to put new batteries in my Walkman, and when I looked out again, he was standing on the patio, waving at me. I was so mortified, I sank into the couch. Three minutes later, I snuck a look and he was gone. But I saw him at other times. Sundays, he'd stroll out and read the paper, shirtless, and soak up some sun. We'd wave to each other. One beautiful fall morning, I saw him and his partner laughing as they piled into their red Miata convertible. On the spur of the moment, I imagined, they'd decided to go to Muir Woods or to Napa Valley for a day of wine-tasting. They shuffled with an easiness I envied, like two leaves carried by the same wind. I never spoke to either of them, yet on the day I watched them moving out—box after box after box—I was crushed, as if good friends were leaving town. I wanted to go, too.

I felt like the bad partner at such times—ashamed that I longed for something different, better, easier. I thought it would hurt Steve if he knew. Well, he did know; my moods were transparent. Anyway, Steve wasn't exactly enjoying his new life of disability. He used to say he could handle losing his health "just as long as it doesn't happen too fast," but by the spring of 1995, AIDS had taken off at such a rapid clip it was hard for him to keep up. Years of powerful antiviral medications had caused irreversible nerve damage in Steve's feet, a condition called peripheral neuropathy. The soles of his feet burned red-hot and shooting pains pulsed up his legs, which made it hard for him to walk or stand for long periods, and impossible to go dancing, as he used to. Large doses of antidiarrheals reduced the number of times he had to sit on the toilet yet didn't stop the diarrhea. He'd lost about forty pounds in spite of a four-thousand-calorie-a-day diet. His body was "wasting," as though being eaten up from the inside out by HIV.

Our bed became the center of our apartment, the place where intimacies of the past transformed into long, nakedly honest conversations. Late one night, I'm in bed reading, Steve's up puttering, when he says out of the blue, "Have you ever heard of someone with AIDS dying peacefully?"

"What do you mean?"

"I mean, it's always horrible, painful, isn't it?" Steve kneels on the mattress, giving his feet a rest.

Silence. Images of Peter and Jeff and others. "I don't know. I'm not really sure. Well, yes, it can be."

He leaves to brush his teeth.

Minutes later, Steve returns, begins undressing, and says casually, "You'll have to let me know if you hear about one of those Final Exit seminars." He could just as easily be talking about a garage sale.

"Oh, okay," I say sardonically, "I'll be sure to let you know. Jeez, bub." I smile, put down my book, let out a sigh. "I've been wanting to talk to you about this for a long time. About suicide. I guess I've always known that it might be part of your plan."

Steve gets in beside me. "Yeah, well, wouldn't you feel the same way?"

"Yes, I would. It's just . . ."

"I want to be ready."

"I know, I know. It's not that I disagree with it. With suicide. And I'm not surprised. It's just—I want to be part of the plan, part of the decision-making. Please, include me. I'm afraid you're just going to do it someday."

Steve smiles wickedly. "You mean, like, me saying, 'Good-bye, honey-pie, see you later, I'm going to the Golden Gate Bridge'?"

"Exactly." We both laugh, struck by the absurd turn in the conversation. "I'd follow you right out to the bridge—I'd take a cab if you took our car—and jump off myself."

"No, no, not now. Not yet. Not for diarrhea, for low T cells. If I go blind or get KS or something . . ."

"Yeah, I understand."

I did. Our good friend Carol had lost sight in one eye— and in most of the other—from CMV, an AIDS-related disease that eventually took her. Carol, who was featured in one of my AIDS Foundation media campaigns, possessed both a wraithlike beauty and frailty that drew sympathy, and a toughness and dry humor that deftly refused it. After Carol's death, we bought her barely used car from her husband, and when I drove it alone, I'd sense at times that she was still in the seat beside me.

Toby, a young boy whom we'd met through the AIDS Foundation and befriended, had also died within the past year. When I'd last visited him at home, Toby, age nine, was being treated for just about every serious AIDS-related illness— PCP, CMV, MAI, and a new one I'd never heard of before, PML, a neurological disease. Through holes in his chest, he was hooked up by tubes to a mobile infusion machine that administered different drugs. Resting on a tattered, dirty couch, this feisty boy looked leashed-up, like a small, old, and tired junkyard dog.

Toby lived with his parents and numerous relatives in a tiny subsidized apartment near the Western Addition. It was filthy, infested with cockroaches, and noisy. While I sat with Toby, his father and uncle played cards and smoked cigarettes at a table nearby. The television was turned up so loud, I couldn't hear Toby unless I leaned down toward him. PML had caused paralysis of his right side; his neck couldn't hold his head up. A tiny black kitten pounced onto the couch. "That's Melody," he said. "I got her as a gift from ACT UP." Paralysis had frozen his face into an old man's smirk, but a boy's mischievous delight lit his eyes as he teased the kitty with string. When I later said I had to be going, he gripped my right hand with his left. "It's cold, you're so cold," Toby said. My hand looked huge in his as he blew a whistle of warm air on it.

Steve and I lived at an intersection of faith, directly across from a Catholic church and a Buddhist temple, at the corner of Pine and Octavia Streets. A Montessori school, diagonal from our building, closed the grid. On Sundays, I'd sit on our couch and read the paper, coffee cup on the windowsill. Steve would be asleep in the next room, earplugs thumbed in. At ten-fifteen, car doors would start to slam, as invariably as Montessori kids cried, first thing Mondays, and garbagemen dragged clanging bins over concrete, Tuesdays and Fridays. While people assembled at Saint Francis Xavier Catholic Church, I heard voices—spare, stretched-out voices. With their arrhythmic inflections and unself-conscious ebullience, each word sounded carefully chosen, deeply felt, and often, incomprehensible to me. This was the sound of deaf church.

I'd put down my newspaper. Gathered across the street, standing on the steps, dozens of parishioners clustered. I rarely saw them talking in large groups. In twos or threes, they carefully observed one another as they read lips, interpreted signs, absorbed every subtle facial cue. There appeared to be as many forms of expression as different degrees of deafness: vocal speech, finger spelling, sign language—all combined at times or alternated back and forth—with ringing whoops or cries as punctuation marks.

I had no idea what they were saying, yet it hardly mattered. I was fascinated by their ability to speak with their bodies and hear with their eyes. Most did not use voices, but relied upon arms, hands, and wonderfully expressive faces to give shape to their ideas and feelings. The individuals opposite them paid sharp attention. From my third-floor window, these casual conversations began to seem terribly fragile: if one looked away, one missed something. With smiles and gentle nods, they constantly assured each other, *Yes, yes, I hear you.*

It was this exquisitely refined quality of *listening*, of patiently watching one another, upon which I most loved to eavesdrop. How much is literally spelled out for them? I wondered. How much is left to intuition?

After many Sundays of listening with my own eyes, the language of deaf church became the source of another kind of fascination. It requires faith, it appeared to me, just to communicate. Faith that their thoughts would be understood. Faith in themselves and others. Faith much like that which, week after week, drew them together so wordlessly. I'd watch until the sidewalk emptied. At ten-thirty, the church doors closed, services began, and I returned to the *New York Times,* as I did to my own defenses and questioning.

At thirty-four, I found myself at an intersection, suspended between youth and middle age, between the Catholicism with which I was raised and the nihilism to which I was susceptible, between belief and uncertainty. It was an unnerving position. I felt as though I'd reneged on an oath I'd made to myself at fourteen.

Everyone has their spiritual revelations. Mine occurred while seated in Sister Charatina's eighth-grade course on Greek mythology. I quite suddenly understood one day the meaning and redemptive power of *irony*. Here was this wizened seventy-year-old nun—with her stories of exorcisms as a missionary in China and her sliver of "the True Cross" hanging in a pendant about her neck—teaching the ancient Greek belief system as fairy tales. The next hour, in religion class, she would humorlessly teach the Gospels and prepare us for the Holy Sacrament of Confirmation. Catholicism was all fabulousness and cruelty, an elaborate ruse with a different cast of demons and idols, from that day forward. Yes, I would get confirmed, as was required by my father, attend mass, take Holy Communion, go to confession, and serve obediently as an altar boy. And I would believe *nothing*.

Over the years, I grew so tired of hearing lapsed Catholics, especially gay men like myself, say that, while they cannot abide the doctrine, stand the pope, or fall to their knees in prayer, they "love the Church's rituals, all the vestments and incense, the bloody crucifixes and gorgeous medieval cathedrals." It was as if they were devotees of a sect dedicated to set design, Hollywood frippery, tableaux in pornographic magazines; *something to set your imagination aflame.* To me, worshiping the pageantry only seemed a way to deflect the hardest question: What do you believe?

No matter how hard I tried to ignore it, the question reappeared—in new guises, with new, louder voices—again and again and again. I wondered what had happened to friends who'd died and what could be done to save Steve's life. I wondered what to do with my own guilt, bitterness, and grief. *Nothing* no longer seemed to be the answer. I asked a close friend what he did when he felt such despair. To my surprise, he answered, "I pray."

"You pray." My response sounded a flat echo of his. What I really wanted to say was "Why?" In some essential way, I didn't believe him, though I envied the ease of his answer. Sensing my doubt and bewilderment (or fearing, with due cause, that I was on the verge of a breakdown), he loaned me a book that promised "a new approach" to prayer. I read a few pages, including the glossary of key words and phrases, yet found the language both as childish and as patronizing as the grade-school catechism that I had deplored.

Later, while lying awake in bed, I tried it again anyway. I still wanted to pray—to be able to pray. I couldn't conjure up a God, so I focused instead on an image of Carol. I became distracted by her shy smile, her graceful fingers, her fine blond hair, yet she never spoke, and I couldn't find a voice to whisper a single word to her. Missing Carol, I felt more desolate than when I'd started. Besides, I thought, if she were in a position of divine power, she would help me if she could, as she had in life. Wouldn't she?

I was reminded of an article I'd skimmed in the *Times* several months earlier on prayer's therapeutic benefits. Some group, somewhere, I don't precisely remember, tested the hypothesis that concentrated doses of prayer, administered regularly, improved the health of people with AIDS and other terminal illnesses. Following the rigid standards of federal drug trials, a randomly assigned group of patients was prayed for daily, while a control group received no-prayer placebos over a specified period. The prayed-for "improved," while the not-prayed-for withered slightly.

I didn't find this cheering, any more than the latest report on protease inhibitors—Steve's "next best hope" for an HIV treatment—filled me with unbridled optimism. I thought cynically, we can expect results on prayer's deleterious effects within a few weeks, as always seems to be the case with "promising" AIDS therapies. Resorting to prayer struck me as scraping the bottom of the barrel, a palliative like a shopping spree or a manicure. It won't hurt but neither will it prolong someone's life.

More to the point, the prayer report made me feel manipulated and angry. I had conducted enough experiments of my own over the years to surmise that praying, hoping, or wishing for things seemed like a waste of my limited stores of imagination. I had sent up pleas that my partner might feel a little better. I had bargained for a break—a lower viral load for him, a good night's sleep for me, in exchange for, well, anything—anything. The results were unobservable or contradictory.

As for all that New Age gobbledygook about mind over matter, maintaining a positive attitude, and psychic healing—forget it. I had burned Chinese incense around our bed while Steve meditated. I had been advised one too many times by HIV-negative friends that his plummeting T cells might be "stress-related." And I had placed my faith in enough ineffective drugs and alternative therapies to lead me to one inescapable conclusion: there is no greater hoax of modern science and secularism than the placebo effect.

One evening in the summer of 1995, Steve and I sat opposite one another on our two couches, no TV, no CDs, no sounds off Octavia Street, and I quizzed him about these things. Do you believe in God? Is there an afterlife? Do you pray? Are your prayers answered? Five years together, and we had rarely discussed questions of spirituality.

The deepening shadows raised, rather than concealed, traces of illness on his face. He's lost more weight, I thought compulsively, he looks tired, I shouldn't bother him. Yet he smiled and wryly advised that just because he had AIDS didn't mean he'd figured out the secrets of the universe. "It's not as if, the fewer T cells, the more wisdom. Really, I don't know anything more than you do."

I felt foolish and laughed. Then, effortlessly sweeping away all my anguished metaphysical questions, he said quietly, "You are a good person." There wasn't a hint of mockery or condescension in his voice. He was answering a question I had never bothered to ask. Indeed, he seemed to be saying, this is all I know, all one can know, the only question one need ask about one's life. The rest—whether Catholic doctrine or Buddhist teachings—well, perhaps it is all mythology. As for Carol and all my other dead friends (or God, for that matter), maybe I should expect to hear nothing back if I whisper, in gratefulness or despair, to them. Death may have a whole new language, composed only of eloquent silences. Perhaps now they are simply the listeners, patiently watching me.

~

The Patient

STEVE'S WAKING up earlier was the first subtle sign that his health was improving. As part of a clinical trial, he'd been taking one of the new protease inhibitor drugs, Saquinavir, for about five weeks when, in February of 1996, I noticed a modest change in his daily routine. And in mine. I'd become used to writing until noon on weekends while Steve quietly slept, yet now he was out of bed by eleven. I turned off the computer and joined him for coffee. Over the next few weeks, he appeared to gain a bit of energy. Once or twice, he drove the car by himself. He made a trip back to the gym after six months away. It was he, not I, who woke first some mornings to get his pills.

Ordinariness started to return to our lives, with a bit of

hope mixed in. This strange, new hopefulness was legitimized by an evening phone call from Marge late that month. I happened to answer the phone. "I've got fabulous news," she announced without saying hello, without saying who was calling. "One hundred seventeen T cells and an undetectable viral load."

"Oh my God. Steve?" I handed him the phone. "It's Marge. It's working."

You know that feeling when you've just typed something on a computer, it's incredibly long and important, and your fingers can't move fast enough to click SAVE? You feel as if the computer will betray you and inexplicably crash before your very eyes? Then you save the document twice, three times, just to be safe? Well, I do. And that's how I felt after Marge's phone call. I wanted to freeze time, to preserve that perfect moment—the hint of mirth in her voice, the exultant sense of relief—before bad news and bad blood work returned.

This wasn't the first time Steve's health had improved, surging with a burst of T cells like a sudden updraft of warm air, which shortly thereafter would blow cold. I had to admit, though, this was different. The protease inhibitors, of which Saquinavir was the first of several, effectively disarmed HIV, neutralizing its ability to replicate if taken in a "cocktail" with other treatments. Within a few months, the first protease inhibitors would formally be approved by the FDA and make national headlines, hailed inaccurately in some cases as a "cure for AIDS." Safer and more potent than drugs of the past such as AZT, they did appear to provide a way toward the future—a chance of surviving a fatal disease. Indeed, as Steve's T cells steadily crawled back up in subsequent months, the diarrhea stopped, he started gaining weight, and he felt both more energetic and relaxed.

While protease inhibitors could clearly be credited with Steve's revived health and spirits, the emotional respite they provided allowed another issue to come forth: Why was my insomnia unchanged? In recent years, I'd reflexively attributed it to anxiety about Steve, compounded by pressures in my working life, yet now it was obvious that something more was going on, something else was to blame.

One night late that year, I left bed at 2 or 3 A.M., turned on a small lamp in the kitchen, and began rustling through the cabinet for a Xanax or Ambien or Restoril, whatever I could find of Steve's or mine. When I closed the cabinet door, a pill bottle in hand, I was startled to find Steve standing in the doorway. "What are you doing?" he asked.

"God, you scared me. I'm, I'm"—my voice was edging into defensiveness and, possibly, a lie—"I'm, well, I'm taking a sleeping pill."

"Yeah, I know."

In the awkward silence, I gathered that he'd intended the question more broadly. "I don't know," I sighed. "I really don't know anymore."

Steve did not smile sympathetically, as I wished he would, nor did he go back to bed. He looked serious—and tired himself.

"I can't sleep," I said.

"Well." Steve sat in a kitchen chair. "So?"

I put the pill bottle down and remained standing.

"So what if you can't sleep tonight?" he said. "What would happen? What's the worst thing?"

"God, I have so much to do tomorrow—that essay to finish, an eight-o'clock meeting at work, I'm supposed to meet Lisa for dinner, I haven't been to the gym in a week . . ."

Steve just shrugged his shoulders, let me listen to myself as I rambled on.

I sat down. "I don't want to be tired."

"Do you really think a sleeping pill will help?"

I shook my head. I knew the drug hangover would last till afternoon, at which point ordinary fatigue would set in.

"You *will* sleep," he said simply. "You will. Maybe not tonight. But you will."

This made me smile. It sounded so right and true.

"I'll stay up with you," he said.

Like when we first lived together, I thought.

I put the sleeping pills back in the cabinet as Steve turned off the lamp. "Come on," he said, "let's get in bed."

After I turned thirty-six in January 1997, I gave myself a midlife ultimatum to get a grip on my insomnia. AIDS had taught me that there definitely was a cutting edge of science, but you had to go looking for it. I told my primary-care physician I wanted to see a specialist at the Stanford University Sleep Disorders Clinic—one of the most esteemed sleep clinics in the world. Long out of sleep suggestions himself, beyond hypnotics, he was glad to make the referral. Persuading my HMO, however, took some finagling. Stanford, located in another county, was not a preapproved clinic and the initial visit would cost $264. I'm sure they wanted to be certain I was worth the investment.

"Look, let me put it to you this way," I told a customer service representative after my second request had been denied by the HMO. "If not this, you're going to end up paying for years of psychiatric services."

A week later, the approval letter arrived.

The first available appointment at Stanford was a full month away: a sure sign, if ever I needed one, that I was not alone while awake at night. In fact, I was in good company: "chronic insomnia" (abnormally prolonged sleeplessness) afflicts at least 15 percent of all Americans; "transient" or "short-term insomnia" (lasting a couple days or a couple weeks) bothers about 35 percent. I was just one of 150 million weary citizens.

Steve joined me for the 10 A.M. appointment, to be a second pair of ears as much as to keep me company. I came to the clinic prepared, having completed a 175-point sleep-disorders questionnaire. Naturally, most of the questions were about one's behavior while awake—one's condition while asleep being, by definition, incognizant. They seemed to be plumbing for habits, states of mind, and tendencies to nod off at inopportune times. One question inquired if I sometimes drove my car "to the wrong place," without remembering how I got there. My favorite question, number sixty-four, asked if I found myself "doing things such as writing nonsense instead of notes, or mixing together chocolate and gravy?" *Only in my dreams* was not one of the possible responses. I was hardly surprised by the sleep clinic's address: the Stanford Psychiatry Building.

While waiting to register, I overheard a conversation about the opposite of my problem, someone with narcolepsy: "Well, at least he doesn't fall asleep when he's *driving* anymore," a woman gratefully told a doctor. Clearly, they did more than take away his car keys, I thought to myself. Maybe my sleeplessness will also be cured. My reverie was interrupted by a sleep-staff nurse, who signed me in and, for unknown reasons, took Polaroids of my jawline and face. "Look sleepy!" she said, which prompted the smile she was after.

The waiting room was conspicuously free of disorder. Beige furniture appeared to have sprouted from the beige carpeting. The only magazines were years-old copies of *Shutterbug* and *Purchasing*. Behind glass, shelves displayed thick medical texts such as *Principles and Practice of Sleep Medicine* alongside a setup of a pajama-clad teddy bear in a doll's bed.

Steve picked up a pamphlet titled "Insomnia" and killed time by breaking the word down into anagrams. His first penciled attempt: "I son, I man."

"I impressed," I said.

"Okay, okay. . . . How about 'I am no sin.'"

"Amen." Looking over his shoulder at his scribblings, I offered my own: "'I'm insano.'"

Chuckling to himself, Steve pulled a sci-fi book from his pocket.

Unused to being the patient in a doctor's office, I felt nervous and antsy. With nothing to occupy myself, I replayed in my head a dinner-party conversation from a few nights before. The woman seated next to me confided that her baby-sitter sleeps just three hours a night. "Barbara gets so much accomplished, it's amazing! On top of running a day-care center, she's raising her own three kids and getting a law degree."

Probably training for a marathon, too, I thought. The insomniac's pride in *not* sleeping—equal only to her long list of accomplishments and inhuman fortitude—stung with familiarity. Sleeplessness breeds arrogance; we regard ourselves as members of an elite society. In the end, of course, insomnia exacts its price. "Barbara was finally so tired," my dinner companion continued, "she went to a hypnotherapist." Through regression therapy, she "recovered a memory" of her mother smothering her with a pillow when she was a baby. It didn't kill her but it did leave her permanently sleep-disturbed. "Isn't that remarkable!"

"Yes," I conceded: *remarkable* that you trust an insomniac with unsmothered memories to do your baby-sitting.

Now, glad to be at a medical facility rather than at my own New Age rebirthing, I was even more grateful when a doctor finally called my name and led Steve and me to an exam room.

Dr. Bradley wore a monogrammed white coat and a grave

expression. He volleyed questions in a voice so free of affect that it was filled with darker meanings. "When do you go to bed? Do you read in bed? Watch TV?" That is, *I* filled his voice with meaning. The questioning made me feel like a bad student more than a bad sleeper, and at first I wanted to give him "right" answers rather than honest ones.

I quickly gathered, however, that no fib got past him. If I don't come clean here in this bright office, I thought, I'll give it all up in the sleep chamber. Under polysomnographic evaluation, electrodes planted on my skull will drain me of all my sleep secrets. Computer printouts will chart each toss and turn. A team of sleep scientists will scrutinize my every yawn.

"Are you afraid to sleep?" The doctor's words took the slow path across the room.

I looked at Steve and silently mouthed *afraid,* as if sounding out an entirely unfamiliar term. He pursed his lips; he wasn't going to rescue me.

"I'm afraid . . . of not being *able* to sleep," I said at last, making a clear distinction. "Usually, I start thinking about the night ahead right after waking up."

"How much coffee do you drink a day?" Dr. Bradley asked.

"Three cups. Two or three," which was the truth. "Never after one o'clock," I added, which was not. Steve cleared his throat. Dr. Bradley didn't flinch or glance up from his note-taking; he'll just test my urine sample later for caffeine, I figured. "Actually," I said, breaking down, "sometimes up to five o'clock."

Unbidden, I then confessed to every sleeping pill I'd ever ingested, beginning with the knockout drug at the college infirmary and on through Xanax. Dr. Bradley did not look the least bit shocked.

"Yes, I got a copy of your medical file from your doctor," he informed me.

A knock at the door brought two more white coats into the room: neurologists, there to observe. Indian women of the same height, they could have been twins. One wore eyeglasses, the other a beautiful pair of shoes. His diagnostic interview completed, Dr. Bradley began a physical exam—heart rate, blood pressure, etc.—all very ordinary until I opened my mouth and said, "Aaaaahhhhh."

The doctor's white-blond eyebrows rose. He summoned the neurology twins. One appeared over each of his shoulders—I had a vision of the tiny singing duo in old Godzilla movies—and he lit up my mouth. "Again, please."

"Aaaaahhhhh."

"Hmmmmm," they hummed, all three at once. "A very large *uvula*," Dr. Beautiful Shoes declared, using a word I'd always found vaguely sexual to describe the dangling flesh at the back of the throat.

Dr. Eyeglasses was speechless.

"Yes, it is kind of crowded in there," Dr. Bradley stated. As he poked around my mouth with his Popsicle stick—his face alive with emotion for the first time—I was struck by the thought that doctors must *become* doctors because they're fascinated by the human body, especially its peculiarities. "A big uvula, a steep, narrow palate, a tongue that's a bit too big for your jaw—see how its edges are scalloped?" He looked positively ecstatic. "Do you snore a lot?"

"No."

"Yes," Steve interrupted. All eyes turned to him. "Well, lightly," he demurred.

"You'll snore more loudly when you get older," Dr. Bradley said. "Especially if you gain weight. You know—if you get a fat neck."

I got the picture. It was a snapshot of my deceased grandpa Herbert: 280 pounds. "That's not currently part of my fitness plan."

"Good," Dr. Bradley said, sitting down again, "because you are a prime candidate for obstructive sleep apnea." He looked pleased with himself, having formulated both a prognosis and a diagnosis.

Technically speaking, my fat uvula predisposed me to sleep apnea, but not the rest of me. I had been at the same lean weight for twenty years. I exercised religiously, walked to work, and didn't smoke. I still took a drink on occasion, but was far too "hypervigilant," as the doctor correctly assessed, to overeat or overdrink. As a matter of fact, these were precisely the qualities that contributed to my classic American sleep disorder.

"You have psychophysiological insomnia," the doctor pronounced. I was the kind of person who worried about the quantity and character of my sleep, not to mention the precise wording of my diagnosis: I asked him to say it again while I lip-synched and memorized it.

"Insomnia is part of your psychological makeup," he explained, a tendency I likely developed as a young boy, just as others assume propensities for headaches or weight gain. Disturbed sleep is a sign of unrest—of stress, anxiety, depression, and other side effects of everyday living. It allows the mind to express itself in a way that cannot be ignored. I am also unusually sensitive to changes in my body's clock, such as those caused by jet lag or, for that matter, by sleeplessness. Insomnia will come and go throughout my life, he added: "There isn't a cure."

Tissue paper covering the exam table crinkled like old parchment as I leaned back against the wall. I was unexpectedly satisfied with this news: incurable and therefore *not crazy*. It wasn't so much that I'd failed to respond to the years of prescription drugs and other remedies, as it was that they'd failed to work for me. This was not an admission of powerlessness, but clarity about the peculiar relationship of my mind to my body. It all made perfect sense. Still, I was left with one un-avoidable fact: many nights I couldn't sleep.

"So, what can I do?"

Psychophysiological insomnia was neither serious nor mysterious enough to warrant a night in the sleep chamber, monitored by polysomnography. As therapy, Dr. Bradley pre-scribed a number of behavioral techniques for "improved sleep hygiene," such as composing a "worry list" before going to bed, and getting out of bed if my worries kept me awake for more than twenty minutes. Among the most effective measures, he claimed, was an oddly primitive one. I was told to get out of bed at the same time every day and expose myself to as much light as possible for thirty minutes. In lieu of full-strength out-door sunlight, he recommended a $200 light box that emitted ten thousand lux (artificial indoor lighting is not bright enough). The aim was to recalibrate my circadian clock. I was to do this for six weeks before returning for a follow-up exam: turn on the lamp or take a walk, even before making coffee. "Caffeine may jump-start the body," he explained, "but it's sunlight that triggers your internal clock." With daytime distin-guished from nighttime, sleeptime would come more naturally. The doctor concluded grandly, "We are trying to re-create the dawn!"

⁕

Maybe this will actually work, I told myself, as Steve and I walked from the cool, sterile environment of the sleep clinic into the noon sun. In the parking lot, I stopped before getting into our car, turned my face up to the clear sky, eyes closed, and then opened them wide, letting them water as the sun momentarily burned my irises—a direct shot to my brain, like a long swallow of tequila straight from the bottle. "Ahhh, med-icine," I said, beaming, settling in behind the wheel of our

Saturn. Then, on second thought: "Steve? I think you'd better drive." By the time we reached the freeway, my field of vision had mostly stopped dancing with purple sunspots.

Re-creating the dawn was one thing. Reprogramming my mind at bedtime, I knew, would prove more challenging. Exactly as Dr. Bradley directed, I sat in our living room at ten-thirty that night, on the dot, lights dimmed. My head was bowed over a fresh yellow legal pad positioned in the center of my cleared desk, like a fetish object radiating talismanic powers. Pen in hand, I began calling up all of my worries as I prepared to put them to paper. At once, my head sprung up: "Hey, Steve!"

He appeared in the doorway, a toothbrush spiking a patient smile.

"Just for clarification: Did Dr. Bradley say to list the things I have to *do* or the things I'm *thinking* about, because if it's all the things—"

"Ev'r'th'ng," he mumbled through toothpaste foam.

"Everything," I repeated. "Gotcha. Thanks."

Returning to my task, I started at the top of both the page and my head: "Sleep," underlined, was my first concern. "Get some." That sufficed—short and sweet, like a grocery list. "Work" came next. In the same way that farmers rotate their crops to replenish the soil, I changed jobs every couple of years. I'd recently gone back to the San Francisco AIDS Foundation, where I was in charge of individual fund-raising. I detailed the next day's agenda—meetings to attend, phone calls to make, etc., everything that floated to the surface. That completed, I turned to my freelance writing, to household chores, to personal phone calls and letters, and to "Miscellaneous," an omnibus for spare troubles. Naming and articulating each of these, I found, added an extra veneer to the anxieties themselves, until the canary-yellow page was clogged with black worries. It was quite humbling—in truth, even a little humiliating—to see all my cares and woes spelled out. In my head, they thrived like yeast in sugar water, heating up and expanding, bubbling with ripe, organic life. But on the page, they were rendered inert, flat, a little silly.

Finished at 10:55, I put the worry list away, joined Steve in bed, and picked up a book. Technically speaking, reading in bed was an infraction—the bed was to be used only for sleeping and sex, Dr. Bradley prescribed. I was not to watch TV in bed, work in bed, eat in bed, or even have long, involved conversations with Steve in bed. The idea was to redefine the bed as a place for sleeping only, pure and simple. But reading, as I told the doctor, was one activity that actually *did* make me drowsy, so a few pages were permitted. However, when my mind soon strayed from the words on the page—as fresh anxieties bubbled up—I closed the book and left bed, again as Dr. Bradley suggested. I added these new items to my worry list, which was relegated to the other room, as before, behind a closed door. The symbolism was simplistic, yet the exercise was amazingly effective. As long as they were penned into another room, the anxieties could not invade the bed. When I resumed reading, I became authentically sleepy. The last thing I recall is saying "Good-night."

Over the following six weeks, my nightly list grew shorter and shorter until, by the time I returned to Stanford for my follow-up appointment, I no longer needed one. I trained myself to put things aside mentally when I was ready to sleep. And if I couldn't, I got out of bed, went into another room, and wrote them down. On nights when I truly wasn't drowsy, I also took advantage of Dr. Bradley's simple directions for the correct way to take a sleeping pill such as Ambien: early. Rather than waiting until the middle of the night, nip insomnia in the bud by taking a hypnotic as early as possible. And never take them for more than three or four nights consecutively; otherwise, one becomes dependent on them. I woke at the same time every day, even on weekends, as instructed; took a walk to expose myself to morning light (I didn't bother with the light box); and eliminated caffeine after one o'clock.

I can't say for certain that the *amount* I slept changed, yet my view of sleep gradually did. I came to feel, more often than not, that I was in control of sleep rather than controlled by sleeplessness. In the nightly tug-of-war, I held a slight edge. Perhaps it goes without saying, but I feel obliged to add that this reversal made me unequivocally glad. It's recently come to my attention that not all patients who leave sleep clinics with a clear diagnosis, or maybe even a "cure," end up being happy about it. For some, such as Rhonda Gilmore, a forty-year-old technical writer living in Indianapolis, disordered sleep is still "normal" and normalized sleep is a new disorder.

Rhonda, with whom I had a series of conversations by telephone and through E-mail, had long known that her sleep was "different from other people's." It was the punch line to a story her mother often told. When Rhonda was an infant, her parents lived in a tiny one-room apartment in university housing for married students. Her father brewed homemade beer, and the only place to store fresh cases was under the bassinet. He put too much sugar in one batch and later, while Rhonda slept, a whole case blew up—bottle tops shooting off as if a firing squad were under her bed. "After that," Rhonda told me with a laugh, "I never slept through the night." According to her mother, Rhonda would stop breathing during sleep, as though scared to death, in what sounds like an apneic episode. Her mother would shake her until Rhonda caught her breath again. By the time she reached high school, Rhonda's roof-rattling snoring, screaming in her sleep, sleeptalking, sleepwalking, and crazy dreams had become the stuff of family legend.

Today she's the mother of a twenty-two-year-old son and a seventeen-year-old daughter, and Rhonda recently married the man she's lived with for ten years, Don. It was he who "ratted" her out about her "bizarre sleep," she explained. About eight years ago, she had to see her general practitioner for an unrelated problem. Don joined her at the appointment and, to her horror, blurted out to the doctor that her snoring could not possibly be normal. (To give me a sense of just how loud her snoring can get, Rhonda noted that Don is "completely deaf in one ear and mostly deaf in the other." What's more, the two of them work at home and keep separate bedrooms. On different schedules, Don was always up late working in his room while Rhonda slept in another. Even through two closed doors and with a severe hearing loss, he could still hear her "choking and snoring and making a huge amount of noise.")

While she knows that Don was only concerned for her health, Rhonda can't hide her continuing resentment. Her sleep would never have changed had Don not tattled to her doctor, who in turn sent her to a sleep-disorders clinic in Albany, New York. It took just a one-night stay in the laboratory, hooked up to a polysomnography machine, to diagnose Rhonda with a severe case of obstructive sleep apnea syndrome (OSAS), a disorder her father also had. Incredibly, Rhonda stopped breathing and woke up 113 times during that single night. By comparison, an average, healthy person would never stop breathing during sleep and might wake up briefly, at most, four or five times. Even though sleep apnea is twice as common in men, recent research shows that women with the disorder have a higher mortality rate, which may mean they're more susceptible to OSAS risks such as hypertension. In Rhonda, the physicians detected serious oxygen depletion. Her condition, at age thirty-two, was life-threatening.

When Rhonda was given her diagnosis, the physicians showed her a video they'd recorded of her apneic episodes while sleeping. "It was horrific," she admitted to me. "Dreadful. I can understand now why Don was so alarmed."

She later returned to the Albany clinic to be fitted with a CPAP (continuous positive airway pressure) machine, a portable bedside unit with a breathing mask that forces air into the nose during sleep, keeping the passages open. While people with OSAS may alternatively use dental devices that keep the airway open or undergo major surgery to remove the uvula and parts of the soft palate, CPAP (pronounced "see-pap") remains the most common treatment. Using it for the first time, Rhonda stayed overnight at the sleep laboratory. Everyone but her was pleased with the results.

"It was like walking into a totally black closet and then immediately walking out again, except it was eight hours later," she recalled. "It was one of the weirdest and most disconcerting experiences of my life. I was used to being aware of my dreams, aware of my environment while I slept, aware of time passing. And with CPAP, there's nothing. It's like turning to Channel Zero.

"Even after several years of using it, I still find it peculiar. I admit that I probably function better when I use the machine regularly, but it is still a disturbing kind of sleep to me. I have this vague sense of being cheated."

I pointed out that, to most people, Rhonda's "black closet" time would be a perfectly blissful, uninterrupted night's sleep. "But it doesn't feel *right*," she insisted. "It feels *terribly* unnatural!

"I don't have any dreams at all with CPAP. Rather, I don't remember them, because I sleep so deeply. There are no more pictures, no more strange stories. There are also no more nightmares, which is kind of nice. But in the past I've had good insights from my dreams and I don't like to lock them up, where I can't get to them."

Rhonda confessed that OSAS often left her feeling terribly fatigued and that she is more prone to illnesses than most people, such as yearly bouts of pneumonia. And yet, like a closet smoker sneaking a cigarette, she still indulges in her dreamy apneic sleep a couple nights per week, much to the irritation of her husband. She can go for about four days using CPAP, she told me, but then her will collapses. In part, this has to do with the discomfort of wearing the apparatus. It dries out and irritates the nasal passages; she wakes feeling as if she has a sinus infection.

There is one possible long-term alternative both to using CPAP and to getting surgery for OSAS: losing weight. I was curious to know how much weight doctors have suggested Rhonda lose, but she deftly avoided answering me. While being overweight may not have initially caused sleep apnea—it's possible she's had it since infancy, the result of the anatomical structure of her throat—it likely contributes to its severity. But she has not succeeded in shedding any pounds. Deeply resistant to trading in her familiar sleep, Rhonda seemed afraid of losing a facet of her identity.

"I'm also a little suspicious of the science," she explained. In her mind, "a quote-unquote normal night's sleep" is not the cure-all that doctors and others would have you believe. "Part of the lure of sleep-disorders literature is in promising you this kind of magical potion: sleep. As if it were a drug—something that will make you feel better and *be* better, turn you into Superman. And it turns out, of course, not to be the case." Sure, she might get eight hours' sleep, but in the morning she is the same person, in the same body, in the same situation: "a sleep weirdo," as Rhonda referred to herself, as she was as a baby and will always be.

Her perspective jibes with my own to a degree. I have a simple theory that people are wired like digital alarm clocks. If a clock is unplugged and then you plug it in again or if there's been a power outage, its memory is wiped out, the numbers flash: 12:00, 12:00, 12:00, 12:00 . . . You have to fiddle with the buttons on the back to set the correct time: hour, minutes,

A.M., P.M. Backward, forward. Then you have to reset the alarm—press that while pushing this. You might have to pull out the operating instructions to get the damn thing back to normal.

People come equipped with similarly aggravating circuitry. At birth, an intrinsic self clicks on deep within the central nervous system: "human noon," as I think of it. Maybe it's not housed in the brain, but behind the knees or at the crook of the neck—a ticklish, thin-skinned place. Flourishing in darkness, it's molded into a basic shape during childhood. I don't know how, of course, but I can tell you this: the Human Genome Project is not going to reveal it. We are not purely products of heredity.

Later in life, when our bodies or psyches get knocked off track, we may default to an earlier setting. We cry or fuss or pout or go dumb, overeat, sleeptalk, sleepwalk, or as in my case, can't sleep. It is inevitable, no matter how much we think we've grown or worked out issues in therapy. At our most vulnerable, our most exhausted or stressed-out or anxious, we revert to human noon, for a flash at least, like that digital 12:00 preset at the factory.

I'm not suggesting that our most basic responses are all set in childhood and thereafter unchanging. Nor that they are all signs of weakness. There are also default settings for positive traits—inner strength, optimism, happiness—our selves at our best. And we do assume new traits as a result of adult experience. As Steve regained his health, for example, he didn't concurrently recover a sense of himself as "healthy." Healthier, yes, but not healthy. That memory was wiped out forever. Even after he rebuilt his body—leaner and more muscular than ever—and his T cells rose higher than they'd been in seven years, taking him far away from the "land of AIDS," he could never return to where and who he'd been before, HIV-positive—asymptomatic. He would always be, technically and otherwise, a person with AIDS who'd come close to death. If nothing else, the drugs he had to take unfailingly seven times daily reminded him. More importantly, appearances to the contrary, he still *felt* disabled. The nerve damage got progressively worse, oddly enough, rather than better. Given his otherwise good health, it was confounding to Marge, who in March of 1998 sent him to a neurologist.

Her name was Dawn. I took that as a good sign. She had blond hair and a gold-capped front tooth, which glinted through her soft, narrow smile. With Steve's permission, five doctors visiting from Japan observed silently as Dawn McGuire, M.D., performed a neurological exam. She tested his eyesight, his reflexes, his memory, his balance, and his diminished sense of touch. As she worked, she spoke to the doctors about his case in clinical language that Steve and I scarcely understood, but she touched him like a concerned friend. She protectively held her hand over his, for example, as she described the advanced peripheral neuropathy that had numbed his feet and turned his hands into red, swollen claws. Dawn said that, with his AIDS history, none of Steve's symptoms were grossly unexpected, yet she had a wild hunch she needed to rule out; Steve would have to get a brain MRI. At the close of the appointment, one of the observing doctors, a woman, walked across the room to give me a gift: an origami swan I'd watched her fold during the examination. I was touched by her gesture and unsettled by it: Did she know something that we didn't?

As with nearly all patients who get MRIs, the attendant offered Steve a sedative before the procedure. Some people get frantically claustrophobic while encased for thirty minutes or more in the tomblike MRI machine with its loud jackhammer noise. Characteristically, Steve declined. Later he told me he'd closed his eyes and imagined it was a sunny day and he was standing on a street corner near a crew doing roadwork. He also added that it was such an awful experience he knew that something had to be wrong. "Dawn wouldn't have put me through that just for the hell of it."

I heard the shower running when I got home from work two days later. I'd just shut the door when Steve turned the shower off and called out for me to come into the bathroom. He sounded displeased. I thought to myself, what's he pissed about? As he pulled back the shower curtain, I saw that his body was pink from the hot water and his face was pale gray. "I have a brain tumor," he spit out as his eyes filled with tears. I grabbed his arm, as though to stop us both from falling. "Dawn left a message. They have to remove it." I felt sick to my stomach as a wave of adrenaline instantly pulsed through me.

Steve's nakedness added to the dreamlike quality of this news. He looked exceptionally beautiful at that moment—his body glistening, muscles taut, nipples erect. In any other circumstance, I might have stripped off my clothes and joined him in the shower. I kissed him lightly on the lips, then we stared at each other in shock until I noticed he was shivering. "Turn the shower back on," I told him, trying to gather my wits. "Warm up."

It was the longest shower I've ever heard Steve take. After he dressed, we sat at the kitchen table and listened to Dawn's answering-machine message and then spoke to her by phone. Her voice was alarmingly calm as she explained that Steve had a pituitary gland tumor, a rare condition called acromegaly. She said it had nothing whatsoever to do with AIDS.

"Just a lucky coincidence, huh?" Steve said. "Not one life-threatening condition, but *two!*"

"I'm afraid so," Dawn replied. After a pause, she added,

"While it's almost certainly a benign tumor, it's positioned right behind the optic nerves, which could be dangerous to your eyesight if not removed. It's made the neuropathy worse because it forces the pituitary gland to flood your body with huge amounts of growth hormone—the last time you needed that much was at puberty. It's like your body's getting the message to *grow*, but there's no room. All the nerves are inflamed. Of course, that's also why you've gotten so muscular—it's like pure steroids." Further, she explained, the excess growth hormone could cause high blood pressure or a heart attack. "I've already started arrangements for your surgery. They won't have to crack open your skull; they'll go up through your mouth. One of the best neurosurgeons in the country is going to do it: Charles Wilson."

Dr. Wilson was as taciturn and cool as Dawn was expressive and comforting. At a brief appointment the week before surgery, I asked him to explain the whole procedure to us. A small, chiseled man in his late sixties, he leaned back in his chair, dark eyes twinkling, and said slowly, "Steve will check in. We'll put him to sleep. A few hours later he'll wake up, and the tumor will be gone." I laughed tightly, both irritated by his condescension and impressed by his self-confidence. There were serious risks, he stated, blindness being one, yet that had never happened under his care. In his busy practice, he often performs four brain surgeries in a day. "I've done thousands." In this instance, I knew, there was a tremendous advantage to Steve's being treated like a statistic.

The presurgery area was a large, cold room of stainless steel and linoleum filled with padded gurneys, each surrounded by a curtain. I had the impression of being inside a huge refrigerated meat truck. Steve dressed in a surgical gown and got under the single white sheet, shivering. We were chatting in the early-morning quiet, as if the truck were in park, idling, when all of a sudden everything went into high gear. In a commotion of efficient activity, the anesthesiologist arrived along with two nurses. They took Steve's vital statistics, reviewed the numerous consent forms, and plunged two IV needles into his arm. I turned around to put his belongings into my bag, and already they were wheeling him off to surgery. I hastened to follow, and with a quick wave, he was gone.

While I'd certainly considered the possibility of losing him to illness before, that was the single most frightening moment: seeing him whisked away on a gurney, his life in others' hands. What if he never woke up? Or instead, awoke blind or brain-damaged?

Five hours later, Steve came out of anesthesia in his hospital room, flanked by nurses, his face bandaged. I tried comforting him with a nervous babble of encouragement as he found himself vomiting blood he'd swallowed during surgery. His immediate response: "Shhhhh. Stop talking." I had to smile. His mental capacity and speech were certainly unharmed. Dr. Wilson later confirmed that the surgery had been successful and he expected no complications.

That night, the hospital's neurology ward was a Grimms' fairy-tale forest of strange noises: moans and screams from other rooms; unplacable gurgling sounds, as if bodies were turned inside out; the frequent clatter of a metal cart pushed by an attendant. The night nurse was a wicked witch, a tiny elderly woman with a heavy Eastern European accent. She roughly took Steve's blood pressure and temperature. I told her that I'd be staying overnight. "No. Not allowed." Her nametag read "Lucretia." Perfect, I thought. My private evil wish that she should be vanquished was apparently granted. At 1 A.M., a new nurse appeared, a peppy, young vision of good health named Kim. She gently changed Steve's bandages and brought me pillows and a blanket.

Steve was in a lot of discomfort, but I found that I could ease him to sleep for a short time by rubbing his feet. Whatever sleep I had stored in me I pictured emptying out through my hands, streaming into the soles of his feet, and up to his brain. Soon, his eyes closed and he was exhaling heavily through his mouth.

Around four o'clock, I arranged three pillows end to end on the floor and positioned myself on top of them. Wearing my coat, I pulled a blanket over me. I could see under his bed and out into the hallway. Fuzzy shadows approached before figures walked past. I heard Steve's wheezing. He's gonna be okay, I told myself, don't worry. Next thing I knew, I opened my eyes. I had fallen asleep and it was morning.

Chapter 18

Final Sleep

AUGUST 19, 1999: I wake to a ringing phone. A glance at the clock: 6:30 A.M. *Ugh.* The only thing worse is waking to screaming. *Brrringgg.* In my half-asleep mind, I test the caller: if it's important, you'll leave a message. Third, fourth ring—a hang-up just as the machine kicks in. *Of course:* a wrong number. Fifteen minutes later, the phone wakes me from a lovely, light hypnopompic interlude, instantly vaporized. *Who the hell?* Now I'm pissed. I look over at Steve, who's got earplugs in, which makes me pissed at him. Again, a hang-up. In fifteen minutes, it's ringing again. Dread overtakes irritation: *Oh my God,* I think, *something's wrong. Someone's died. An accident?* Names start running through my head as I dash for the phone, heart racing.

"Bill?" It's my friend Steven.

"Hey, are you okay?" I answer. "Is Garth okay?"

"We're fine. It's Nathaniel Kleitman."

"*Kleitman?*"

"He's dead. Died on Friday. Friday, the thirteenth. It's in the *Times* today. I've been trying to fax it to you—"

"Christ, the fax wasn't on. That's why—the phone."

"Did I wake you up?"

"Huh? No. No, no, no, no." Why, I think abstractly, must one always *deny* having been asleep when awakened by a phone? Why not flaunt it? You'd think he asked if I'd been drinking at 7 A.M.

"Do you want me to try faxing it again?"

"No, no, I'll go get a paper. Thanks."

My first thought as I begin making coffee: Dr. Kleitman would delight in people being awakened by news of his death.

Without wakefulness, sleep cannot be said to exist.

This brings a smile to my lips.

"Nor can I without caffeine." I toss an extra scoop of coffee into the filter—what the hell, might as well get really wired—and run out to buy a copy of the *New York Times*.

He leads the day's obituaries; four columns above the fold: "Nathaniel Kleitman, Sleep Expert, Dies at 104." Seeing it in print, I feel mildly surprised; I'd begun to think he might outlive me. But there's no doubt, my Hypnos has met his Thanatos. The *Times* runs two photos. One's from Mammoth Cave, 1938, in which he is tinkering with motility equipment beside a raised bed containing Bruce Richardson, who's asleep. Bearded, dark- and scruffy-haired, and wearing a hooded sweatshirt, this forty-three-year-old Kleitman is unrecognizable from the bespectacled sixty-six-year-old in the second picture, a formal head shot. With a crown of silver hair, unsmiling, he is the image of a buttoned-down scientist and patriarch, indeed "the father of contemporary sleep research," as the *Times* commemorates him.

This grim visage contrasts with the final impression left by his obituary. Noting that Dr. Kleitman had participated in many symposiums on sleep in the four decades since his retirement, the article closes with the fact that he gave one of his last public lectures at the 1995 meeting of the Associated Professional Sleep Societies (APSS). Attendees celebrated his one hundredth birthday and, as a colleague recalled, "He was treated like a rock star."

Having recently returned myself from this year's APSS meeting, held at the end of June in Orlando, I have trouble coaxing forth an image of a roaring throng of sleep scientists cheering Nathaniel Kleitman. I try to picture an undulating sea of Itty Bitty Book Lights lifted in a darkened auditorium at the close of his speech four years ago on "Why Infants Wake Up to Nurse"; the centenarian himself returning to the stage for an encore, a rare reading, say, from one of his first published works, 1934's *Studies on the Possible Intoxicating Action of 3.2% Beer;* and concession stands selling T-shirts emblazoned with Kleitman's face and the words SLEEP GOD. All to no avail. My general impression of the attendees was of a deeply serious, conservative group.

The first organized sleep conference was held in 1960 with all the sleep researchers in the world—a total of twelve. At the 1999 APSS conference—a joint meeting of both the Sleep Research Society and the American Sleep Disorders Association—there were thirty-one hundred. A journalist on a press pass, I listened to experts present findings on everything from "Dreams of the Depressed" to "Narcoleptic Doberman Pinschers." Though I hardly needed to duck for all the medical terminology that flew over my head, I also felt that I was among my own kind: men and women as passionate as me about the subjects of sleep and wakefulness.

Out of 561 papers and poster presentations at the five-day conference, over a quarter concerned obstructive sleep apnea syndrome (OSAS). Surgeons brought news of novel techniques for reducing tongue size or trimming the soft palate, while psychiatrists revealed the severe toll that OSAS-related snoring, fatigue, and impotence take on a relationship. Clinicians bemoaned that, though the CPAP breathing machine is effective, compliance is dreadfully low, especially in the long term, because it's so uncomfortable to use. As an alternative, the benefits of a "mandibular repositioning appliance" were touted. At one symposium someone wondered aloud if, in the future, there might actually be a "sleep apnea pill." The comment drew laughs and, I thought, sounded ludicrous until I realized that, in a sense, there already *is* a pharmacological fix: new drugs that help obese people to shed weight, such as the fat-blocker Xenical. Results from a large trial in Sweden showed that apnea symptoms are dramatically reduced if people with morbid obesity lose weight; however, this study was an exception. Though obesity remains the single greatest risk factor for OSAS, advocating weight reduction as even a partial solution was rarely discussed. I was reminded of an AIDS conference I'd attended in Australia in 1997. Convinced that safe sex and clean-needle use were not a long-term solution to ending the AIDS epidemic, some researchers heralded the concept of "prevention technology," which assumed that people couldn't be relied upon to change behavior and that a shot or a pill or a patch was the only hope for preventing HIV. In both settings, I had the disheartening feeling that scientists had given up on the willpower of patients.

Obesity and OSAS are also often culprits in the poor sleep of the elderly, explained Sonia Ancoli-Israel, Ph.D., a researcher from the University of California, San Diego. Many scientists have long believed that sleep deteriorates with age, just as bones become brittle and hair grays; that the need for, say, eight hours' sleep decreases at the same time as the ability to stay asleep wears away. But Dr. Ancoli-Israel—an expert on the sleep of seniors—strongly disagrees. Disordered sleep is not a consequence of age but of other factors, she emphasized, such as apnea, prescription side effects, alcoholism, depression, and circadian abnormalities that are often a result of the living environment. In nursing homes, for instance, her research team found that seniors confined to beds or wheelchairs have little exposure to natural light. Their circadian clocks function almost like those of the blind. Already drowsy from medications and lack of exercise or stimulation, these elderly people constantly doze off during the day and their sleep patterns become fragmented. The damage is not irreversible, Dr. Ancoli-Israel noted. As other scientists have confirmed, older people may produce just as much melatonin as young people. In some cases, nursing home residents' sleep and overall health could be improved simply by taking them outdoors or to a window during the day, and by restricting sleeping to bed and at nighttime.

Still, one must have "some reason for staying awake," as Dr. Kleitman put it in a 1989 interview. That is to say, a reason to live. If one's spouse is deceased, if family or friends are absent, if one is without work to occupy the mind, sleep may be a way to pass time in old age. "Accidentally or intentionally, you take a nap," Dr. Kleitman said. "I watch television—all of a sudden I see a program I had not been viewing. . . . It happens all the time. My wife died twelve years ago, but when she was alive, she would tell me, 'You're asleep!'" Without his wife, Paulena, he pushed himself daily to stay active and alert—to walk to the post office or store. "I make it a point," he said at age ninety-four; "it's like a prescription." One that doubtless helped keep him alive for another ten years.

It had crossed my mind that Dr. Kleitman might actually make an unbilled appearance at the APSS conference. Perhaps I'd spot him on the arms of his devoted daughters, Esther and Hortense. But the closest I came to him was in shaking hands with William Dement, whom Kleitman had referred to as "my prize pupil." Dement had begun working for the senior scientist in 1953 as a University of Chicago medical student. Unlike Eugene Aserinsky, who left the field of sleep science after completing his doctorate, Dr. Dement continued on. In 1963, he took a faculty position at Stanford, where he co-founded the renowned sleep-disorders clinic as well as the medical journal *Sleep* and conducted important early research on narcolepsy and obstructive sleep apnea. Now one of the field's elder statesmen, an amiable, snowy-haired man in his seventies, he is the author of several mainstream books on sleep and a tenured professor at Stanford.

"Nathaniel Kleitman was a really nice person, though very formal, a man of few words," Dr. Dement recalled during a conference discussion on the history of sleep science. "His wife called him Sonny, but to everyone else he was always 'Dr. Kleitman.' " Through hundreds of sleepless nights, the young Dement worked for Kleitman until his retirement in 1960, and they remained close. In his nineties, Dr. Kleitman even became a research subject at Stanford on sleep in the elderly.

In a brief exchange afterward, I told Dr. Dement that I'd been to his sleep clinic and it had been helpful. He looked pleased, as if I'd complimented one of his grandchildren. Already late for his next panel, Dr. Dement rushed off and I wandered into the exhibition hall. Though it contained scores of research poster presentations tacked to bulletin boards, it was primarily a mini–trade show featuring major pharmaceutical companies such as Monsanto, for which the sleeping pill Ambien alone accounts for about half a billion dollars in annual sales. As I made small talk with an Ambien rep, I realized I'd never seen someone so happy at my admission that, yes, I am an insomniac. After giving him an idea of a typical sleepless night, sans Ambien, this big, bluff bruiser of a straight man confessed to "sleeping like a baby, except when I'm on the road and the bed's half-empty." In the awkward pause that followed, there was no mistaking the erotic frisson that rose from two strangers sharing details of how they slept. It would not have seemed out of place to inquire, "And do you sleep in the nude?" Instead, I resumed my tour of the exhibition hall. In booths off to the sides, salespeople hawked various appliances and accoutrements, from gold-plated EEG leads to pricey pillows shaped to minimize snoring. Poor sleep was clearly good for business.

The most eye-catching exhibit featured a large, clear Plexiglas cube that housed a full-size bed on a platform. Tucked into the bed, a young, neatly coifed blond female figure was hooked up to a computerized polysomnograph console—the item for sale. I walked past four or five times, assuming that it was a display mannequin and the brain waves spiking on-screen were simulated. Though she was just eight or ten feet away, she looked too perfect. More to the point, she slept too perfectly—lying on her back, sheets tucked to her chin, arms at her sides, not a wrinkle in the bedspread. Then I saw her chest rise. "My word, is she *real?*" I cried.

"Yup," the salesman chuckled. Thinking back to Armond Aserinsky's story of his simulated REM act as a teenager, I cast a suspicious glance at the computer screen. "See, these are delta waves," he pointed out, reverting to sales mode. "She's in stage four—there's no faking that. The cube's sound-proof."

"Then she's *got* to be drugged," I murmured. Where's that Ambien salesman?

In her eerie, staged tranquillity, the model sleeper literally embodied the phrase *rest in peace*. Moreover, she brought to mind images painted in ancient Egyptian tombs, in which the deceased are portrayed in the bodies they wished to have for eternity—youthful, beautiful—hunting in bountiful fields, mingling with the gods. And perhaps, too, deep in idealized sleep. If heaven *is* as you imagine it to be, I thought as I watched her flawless sleep, then *this* would be my idea of heaven. God knows, it's not how people sleep in the real world.

As evidence, allow me to present United Airlines flight 1623—my trip home from the Orlando conference—a veritable museum of sleep disorders. Seated on the aisle, I, the in-flight insomniac, sip black coffee and keep watch while the specimens sleep. Two seats over, the heavyset, fortyish man propped against the window exhibits every symptom of obstructive sleep apnea. He's so drowsy, he can't stay awake. He tries. He fails. For a moment, I think he might have narcolepsy. Waiting for a beverage, he wakes briefly, but when the flight attendant turns away, his head falls onto a shoulder, rolls down to his chest, and he falls silent, stops breathing. *One, two, three,* I count, like a referee in a boxing match . . . *ten, eleven seconds.* KO'd by his own breath, he chokes, his head snaps back, and he begins snoring.

The small, skinny woman in the row in front of him turns around, kneeling on her seat, to locate the god-awful noise. She takes a long draw off her water bottle, *harumppphs,* then glances at me as if to say, "Look at that disgusting fool!" But now, buckled into her seat, she's snoring, too—a light, congested purr—as is her teenage daughter. The tall, lean man next to me falls asleep after drinking a Dewar's on the rocks. I watch his closed eyelids, looking for signs of REM, but it's too soon. Still in stage 2, I figure. The businessman across the aisle sleeps with mouth agape, his tongue smacking like a dog eating peanut butter. The elderly couple behind him snooze quietly, as does the young, bearded fellow at the opposite window. I look around: every passenger is asleep, six miles above the earth, at eleven-thirty in the morning. What do they pipe into this dry air?

I close my eyes, turn up the volume on my Walkman, and think through my five days at the sleep conference. In retrospect, the most powerful moment occurred the first morning, at the opening ceremony, 8 A.M., Monday, June 21. A thousand chairs filled the Marriott's immense Crystal Ballroom; placed atop each one was a copy of a two-page article from *Science*, September 4, 1953—an article likely as recognizable to every scientist entering that room as his or her own handwriting. Puzzled by its appearance, I picked it up and settled into my seat.

"Slow, rolling, or pendular eye movements such as have been observed in sleeping children or adults," it began, ". . . have also been noted by us. However, this report deals with a different type of eye movement—rapid, jerky, and binocularly symmetrical."

Scanning the familiar byline—Eugene Aserinsky and Nathaniel Kleitman—I glanced up and saw their faces: a photo of them together, projected repeatedly onto three enormous screens at the front of the room. As I strained to understand the meaning of all this, the APSS conference opened with a quick announcement: there would be a minute of silence in memory of Dr. Aserinsky, who had died eleven months earlier. Without stating the obvious, it was implied that his verification of REM sleep and the *Science* paper had launched the modern age of sleep research. The recognition for Dr. Aserinsky, who had felt cheated of his one chance at prominence, was remarkable. I imagined his voice in my head: *Thank you.* This is proof of life after death, I thought to myself: a minute of time devoted to picturing and remembering a man in his absence.

∼

One month later, I was on another flight, bound for Spokane and my twentieth high school reunion. The older I get, the more I fear flying. I find myself preoccupied by a frightful notion: I am going to go *out* the same way I came *to* consciousness: on an airplane. A poetic ending but statistically doubtful. Unlike the afterlife, which I think is largely a product of one's own conception—if you believe in "a better place," then you'll go there—an accidental death is in the hands of the Fates, who write a blacker type of poetry. I'll probably get hit by a Coke truck.

Simple curiosity brought me back for the reunion. It wasn't to see my closest high school friends, with whom I've stayed in touch, but more to see those I secretly idolized or feared as a teenager. What had become of Julie Manor, the magnetic, wild stoner, or of Mike McDonough, the football player on whom I had a crush? And what would they make of me? I possessed none of this curiosity at the ten-year mark; I had ignored the reunions until now. Buoyed by a margarita and the companionship of Teri and three other high school friends, I floated into Gonzaga Prep for the first time in twenty years on a warm Friday night in July. The festivities had just started. We all split up and agreed to share notes later.

The enormous gym was lit as brightly as it would be for a basketball game, but the bleachers were pressed into the wall and a hundred people swarmed around two kegs of beer. I checked in and received a nametag together with a large photo-button of my senior-class picture, a gauzy portrait in which I had lots of feathered hair. Oh, dear. What *did* happen to him? I slipped the button into my pocket and headed for the keg. Some classmates looked so different it would have been easier to recognize them by their laughter, which was un-

changed and in large supply. Names were phrased as wild
guesses—"Rose? Rose Presley? Is that you?"—even when
reading directly from the neatly printed tags. Whether or not
we remembered each other well, no one had qualms about revealing details of his or her personal and professional life, a
liberty that had nothing to do with alcohol.

Half the class of 250 attended, yet neither Julie nor
Mike showed up. Only a few of us had come from out of
town. Early on, I was sure that I had spotted another gay man
in the crowd: he had a shaved head, a pierced ear, and heavily
muscled arms painted with tattoos. He would've looked at
home in a San Francisco leather bar. Cool, I thought. And yet
when I finally ended up talking with him, an alumnus I'd
never known, I realized at once that he was a Harley-riding,
hunting-and-fishing "man's man" from northern Idaho, not the
Castro Street facsimile. His story fit his image: married twice,
a slew of kids, a job on an assembly line at Industrial Park.

For a few moments, I felt like the only gay man who'd
ever appeared in Spokane. While getting reacquainted with
Rich and Mark, whom I faintly recalled from high school,
Rich asked point-blank, "So, are you gay?"

He was looking for clarification, it seemed to me, nothing more. "Yeah, I am."

"What the *hell* did you ask him?" Mark interjected. I
wasn't sure if he was going to defend my honor or attack it.

"I asked if he was gay," Rich explained simply, "and he
said he was."

I watched both of them, trying to sense where I stood.

"You're *gay?*" Mark asked. It had been a long time since
anyone had asked that question with such incredulity. "Gay?"
he repeated.

As I nodded, Mark asked, "What's *that* like?"

"What's it like?" I laughed. "It's like, it's like . . ." I

thought, how to explain? "It's like your being straight; it's just who and what I am," I finally said. Then, I backpedaled: "You *are* straight, right?"

"Hell, yeah. I've just never met a gay before."

Yes, I'm sure you have, I wish I'd said but didn't. I didn't need to.

"Well, my brother's gay," Rich told me as Mark did a slower double take. "I thought you might be, too." Without further comment, Rich, Mark, and I began talking about our jobs.

I found everyone to be warm and open, more so than I expected. The women instantly knew I was gay without my saying so ("And do you have a . . . *lover?*" Dori, a beautician, asked with a naughty smirk), while the men, in general, wished to first give me a chance to imply that I *wasn't,* as though respecting my privacy.

"Married?" a guy named Dan barked at me. "Any kids?"

"Uh, no," I replied, taken aback. He looked like someone I should be wary of. Ah, what the hell, I thought. "I do have a partner of nine years. His name is Steve."

A long pause as Dan computed this equation. Then, sensibly he said, "Well, that doesn't mean you couldn't have kids, does it?"

Chagrined, I replied firmly, "You're right, it doesn't. We just haven't chosen to do that. How about you? Kids?" At which he shared photos of his three daughters.

The whole crowd seemed to be carrying photos of the same three little girls—blond, ages two to ten—as if duplicate prints had come with their wallets. And every mother and father also had tales of sleepwalking and sleeptalking children, when I quizzed them, plus vivid memories of sleep deprivation as a side effect of having babies. In fact, I quickly learned that many of us shared one thing other than our Spokane roots: insomnia. I was glad to hear that the city now has a sleep clinic.

Chip, a motivational speaker, told me that his insomnia was a consequence of constant traveling, while Kandi, a mother of four, had had a rash of sleepless nights since she filed for divorce. Jason, looking tweaked-out, hovered near the chips and salsa. "I work a night shift," he explained between shaky guzzles of beer, "midnight to eight. Couldn't sleep today. And I have to be at work in two hours."

I was curious if he'd ever used melatonin. Researchers had confirmed just weeks prior that, while taking melatonin for insomnia is pointless (the brain releases more than enough melatonin at night, they found; supplements won't make you more drowsy), it does have an effect during the day, when the pineal gland doesn't normally release the hormone. Shift workers who sleep during the day, I explained, may receive some benefit from low doses, as may travelers adjusting to jet lag.

Jason shrugged off my melatonin inquiry, a perplexed scowl on his face. Maybe he thought I was trying to sell him some.

"Well, do you take anything?" I asked.

"Yeah, to stay awake."

Speed, I guessed. "No, I meant to sleep during the day."

"Nah, I just jack off once or twice. That usually does the trick."

"Good to know. Thank you."

Turning around, I saw Ellen Turner, who looked lovelier and more youthful than she had in high school, an impression owed, in part, to the metal braces now on her teeth. Tall and fit, she looked as if she could play for the WNBA. As we caught up, I mentioned that I'd been doing research on sleep and insomnia.

"Lord, I'm becoming an expert on that," she said. "Sleeplessness."

"You must have kids," I ventured.

"Uh-huh. I had my fifth last year."

"Five? Wow, I'm sure a houseful of kids—"

"It's not that, really. My kids are great. I was diagnosed with ovarian cancer a few months ago, and I had to have a full hysterectomy. So I basically started menopause overnight. I get hot flashes and night sweats—middle of the night and I'm wide awake."

"My God, you poor thing, no wonder you can't sleep." I remembered a report from the APSS conference that said estrogen alleviated insomnia in menopausal women. I asked if she'd tried hormone replacement therapy.

"No, I can't take estrogen because of the cancer. Might make it worse." Ellen smiled good-naturedly. "Maybe once I finish chemotherapy."

I grabbed her hand. "I'm so sorry."

She wasn't looking for sympathy but something else. "Hey," she whispered confidentially, "maybe you know of a good sleeping pill?"

My fear of flying vanishes on flights home. I am irrationally convinced that if the plane's going to go down, it will only be in *leaving* San Francisco, never in returning, as if the city itself has some say in the matter. At the Spokane airport late Sunday afternoon, this false sense of security was made more dubious by the fact that I had to take a rickety, twenty-seat shuttle plane to Seattle before transferring to a 727 bound for SFO.

Several hours later, as I stumbled along the passageway between the aircraft and the terminal in San Francisco, I imagined I was in a decompression chamber for sloughing off fatigue and for pulling myself together in anticipation of seeing Steve—a kind of mental car wash. I tucked in my shirt and popped a piece of gum in my mouth, knowing I'd find him a ways beyond the waiting crowds. And there he was, leaning against a post, a peaceful smile on his face.

"Hey, zombie," he said.

"Hey, bub."

Steve, who reserves public displays of affection for very rare occasions, gave me a long hug and a kiss. "Welcome home."

It was past midnight by the time we walked through our door. The apartment smelled as good and familiar as it felt, in the same way that a favorite pillow scrunches up and molds perfectly to your head night after night. Steve was already falling asleep as I crawled into bed beside him and turned off the reading light. In minutes, his breathing shifted to a slightly heavier note. That sound used to be like a gauntlet thrown down—a stage of sleep I was anxious to match as quickly as possible. But I'd found I liked for him to fall asleep first. It was comforting. Lying on my back, I slowed my breathing to rhyme his. My mind raced at a much faster speed, though, circling back to the previous morning.

I had woken up at eight-thirty, as I usually do on weekends, and staggered out of the guest bedroom of my parents' apartment, to make coffee. Mom and Dad were up, already well caffeinated, and I was unprepared to make lucid, pleasant conversation. Even though they live outside of Spokane now, I'd stayed with them rather than at a hotel in part to save money, yet also with a fantasy that, in the spirit of the reunion, we'd have wonderful heart-to-heart talks—smoothing out all past differences in my brief annual visit.

My coffee hadn't cooled enough to drink before my father and I were bickering at the kitchen table. It started when he announced plans for our day together. "Uh, look," I broke in, "I was going to go see some friends today."

"So you don't want to come see my new office?"

"Well, I'd like to, but not in the next half hour, maybe later—"

"And you don't want to have lunch?"

"I, I don't know. I'm not sure what my plans are."

"Play golf?"

He'd obviously come up with a fantasy scenario, too. "'Golf'? I don't play golf."

"Well, you don't have to be a sorehead."

"Who's being a sorehead?"

I looked at my mother as if to an interpreter for a translation of his speech. "Pat, just leave him alone. Let him wake up."

I would have stalked off to my own room if it still existed. In a dramatic gesture, I grabbed my cup, only to spill some coffee on the table. "Shit!" I cried. Leaving the table to find a sponge, I saw that my parents looked shocked at my curse. It had always been like this, it struck me: Dad anxiously approaching, needling me; me resisting, wriggling away; Mom refereeing; and ultimately each of us feeling bad over what had transpired. "Please," I said, sopping up the mess, "can we start over?"

Mom poured me a fresh cup. "Do you want pancakes?" she asked.

"No, thanks."

"Bacon?"

"Mmm, I don't think so. Coffee's great."

"Muffins?"

"No muffins."

We sat in silence for a long while.

"How'd you sleep?" my father asked in a conciliatory tone.

I smiled. "Lousy."

"Yeah," he said. "Me, too."

Looking directly into my father's face, inches from my

own, I saw his watery, bloodshot eyes and—in a heart-stopping flash—their blue irises. His eyes were not green like mine, as I'd thought for many years. I suppressed an urge to exclaim, "Your eyes are blue! *Blue?*" Could they have changed so with age? No, that's unlikely. When did I first start getting it wrong? When was the last time I'd really looked him in the eye? My father would be turning seventy-five in a couple weeks, and I felt as though I hardly knew him.

I sneaked looks at his face. Now, which one's his blind eye? I found myself thinking as I drank coffee. When I was a boy, there was one sure way to figure it out without having to ask him. Walking, Dad preferred for people to be on his right side, especially kids, where he could see them with his good eye and not trip over them. If you weren't positioned at his right, I recalled, he'd slip over to your left side—a silent reminder of his partial blindness. He never said anything, he just moved. In a different sense, I instinctively learned to accommodate myself to his vision. There was a large part of me I always kept him from seeing, as if I intentionally walked on his blind side. Likewise, when it came to seeing me as I really was, his sight often failed him.

Dad left the table and returned a minute later holding an amber plastic container. "Ever try these?" he asked, shaking it like a toy rattle.

He handed me the bottle, a peace offering in the form of sleeping pills. I didn't recognize the drug's name—an old benzodiazepine, I guessed—and the prescription had expired years before. "No, never have. Does it work well?"

"Oh, I don't know. I suppose it did. Hell," he said with a laugh, "you're not supposed to drink if you take them." As Dad sat down in the chair to my left, he gave me the answer I'd been looking for earlier: the left eye.

"Thanks for the tip," I replied, grinning wryly.

I used to wonder if my father's sleep problems could be

blamed on his one-eyed sight—a biological clock that's perpet-
ually half-unwound. An expert in chronobiology recently convinced me otherwise: one eye compensates when both aren't
working, just as one lung can breathe in place of two. It's not
as if there was a shortage of other possible explanations over
the years, beginning with a wife and six kids to provide for—
there's a week's worth of insomnia right there, multiplied by
fifty-two weeks and three decades from the first day to the last
with a child under his roof. Now, he's on the verge of forced
retirement and a year from the age his own father died.

In any case, what I insist on calling insomnia, he calls a
few lousy nights' sleep. Nothing a stiff drink can't cure. It's all
a matter of perspective; or, more accurately perhaps, of identity. While I may see myself as an agnostic gay insomniac, he
thinks of me as a lapsed Catholic and a practicing homosexual; the last in a long line of Hayes men that includes his distinguished great-grandfather, Thomas, who emigrated from
Ireland to America and fought in the Civil War, having enlisted at Abraham Lincoln's first call for soldiers. I will not
marry, have children, and pass on the family name, which is a
source of disappointment to my dad. But there is another way
to look at it. As his only son, I can rest assured, our insomnia
ends with me.

A new night with the same old problem: I leave our bed and
creep into my office. Pulling the blinds up, I move a chair to
the window, then rest my bare feet on the sill, watching for
movement down below. Not a soul is out nor a sound made.
All appears peaceful at three in the morning.

Sensitivity to pain is said to be highest at this hour. If
you're awake, distractions fall away, I suppose, leaving nerves
inflamed, wounds throbbing. Amazingly, dreaming offers a

genuine escape from physical pain, a fact that comforted me in the past and will again, I'm sure, as Steve and I grow older. Even people with chronic, severe pain during the day are numb to it in REM—this is the most persuasive argument that dreaming represents a separate biological state, one that can be explosively visual yet is free of physical suffering.

It sounds like heaven. And in a way, it is. Dreaming led early humans to conceive of a spirit that leaves the body during sleep and travels to fantastic places, which in turn inspired notions of a soul and an afterlife. As it was then, heaven is still widely envisioned as an eternal good dream. Hell's both a nightmare and, as Dante imagined the Inferno, a never-ending state of sleeplessness.

I have trouble conceiving of anything believable in the great beyond. My mind's still littered with images of a cloud city overrun by deceased family pets. "Remember what it was like *before* you were born?" Steve said to me not long ago. He paused as I puzzled. "That's what it'll be like after we die." I don't know where he came up with that, but I find it reassuring.

It's coming up on four o'clock, the very worst time to get a phone call—death occurs most frequently from 4 to 6 A.M. It's as if the old, injured, or ill body, sustained by sunlight, runs out of juice just before dawn. The circadian clock unplugs itself. Lungs collapse. The heart stops. But it's also when most people are sound asleep, so if you were to cry out for help, others would be less likely to hear you. Babies are most liable to die from sudden infant death syndrome right about now.

Given that humans, statistically, tend to die when we tend to be born—at night—do we also die, I wonder, *as* we are born—dreaming? Maybe the white light seen by people who die but "come back" is like the leader film in home movies— the bright, clear frames before the familiar pictures begin. Life ends in a final, glorious REM surge.

If so, I hope it's a damn good dream when I go, one of

those extremely rare ones in which all five senses are employed at once: a dream of swimming, say, at a beach on Kauai—a faint taste of briny water, scent of fresh air, waves crashing. Holding my breath, I close my eyes and dive deep.

It's half past four, the time of lowest body temperature. If you're sleeping, this is when you may drowsily pull a second blanket over yourself. If awake, your ability to perform tasks and think clearly is most impaired. It's also when the body's clock is most easily tricked. Turning on a lamp can be misinterpreted by the brain as morning's first light, ruining any chance of returning to sleep. It is best to pee in the dark.

Four-thirty my time is seven-thirty East Coast time; I could call my friend Maurice, a fellow insomniac who's got thirty years on me and is bound to be out of bed by now. I don't see or talk to him often, and when I do, it's as if he's been saving up wise and witty things to share. Are certain older people truly wiser or are they so cranky, tired, and pressed for time that they're able to see things more plainly?

When Maurice last visited, he gave me a good piece of advice, though he didn't realize it at the time. "You know what I do when I can't sleep?" he explained. "I sit up in bed, push the curtains back, and pull up the window shade." Maurice, who's had a run of serious illnesses, including a major heart attack, said he used to feel frightened and anxious when he couldn't sleep, but now appreciates an aspect of it. "The night air makes me feel safe. Real." He inhaled slowly, as though savoring a whiff he'd brought with him. "I'm not afraid to die. The one thing I will miss most, though, is air at night—life, coming through the window."

I crack open the window onto Octavia. The draft of cold air raises goose bumps on my skin, a shiver. I hear an ambulance far down Pine. Lights flicker on in the California Street apartment building: signs of life. I leave the window open and go climb back into bed with Steve.

ACKNOWLEDGMENTS

THIS BOOK comes with a deep debt of gratitude to my agent, Wendy Weil, and to my editors at Pocket Books, Nancy Miller and Tracy Behar. Special thanks are due also to their assistants, Emily Forland, Anika Streitfeld, and Brenda Copeland, as well as to the experts who aided in my research, including Armond Aserinsky, Robin Chandler and the Special Collections staff of the UCSF Library, Lynne Lamberg, and Margaret Poscher.

I am grateful to Steven Barclay, Sally Ede, Anne Lamott, and Lisa Michaels for their advice and encouragement and to Kathryn Mayeda for her unwavering faith. My deepest thanks as well to Maurice Sendak for his generosity, friendship, and wicked humor.

Had I asked, my partner Steve Byrne really would have given me an hour of his sleep if it were possible. Instead, he patiently edited every line of every draft; helped knock down each wall I hit; and freely supplied large doses of logic, many fearless metaphors, and a great title. I could not have written this book or gotten a grip on my sleep demons without his love and support, for which I remain profoundly thankful.

REFERENCES

⬿

GENERAL

THE FOLLOWING sources are used repeatedly through the book. References for individual chapters are listed below.

Aristotle. *Parva Naturalia*. Translated by J. I. Beare. Oxford: Clarendon Press, 1908.

Arkin, Arthur M., John S. Antrobus, and Steven J. Ellman, eds. *The Mind in Sleep: Psychology and Psychophysiology*. Hillsdale, N.J.: Lawrence Erlbaum Associates, 1978.

Aserinsky, Eugene. "The Discovery of REM Sleep." *Journal of the History of the Neurosciences* 5, no. 3 (1996): 213–27.

———. "Ocular Motility During Sleep and Its Application to the Study of Rest-Activity Cycles and Dreaming." Ph.D. diss., University of Chicago, December 1953.

Aserinsky, Eugene, and Nathaniel Kleitman. "Regularly Occurring Periods of Eye Motility, and Concomitant Phenomena, During Sleep." *Science* 118 (September 4, 1953): 273–74.

Benét, William Rose. *The Reader's Encyclopedia.* 2nd ed. New York: Thomas Y. Crowell Company, 1965.

Binns, Edward. *The Anatomy of Sleep; Or, The Art of Procuring Sound and Refreshing Slumber at Will.* London: John Churchill, 1842.

Bulfinch, Thomas. *Bulfinch's Mythology.* New York: Modern Library, 1998.

Coren, Stanley. *Sleep Thieves: An Eye-opening Exploration Into the Science & Mysteries of Sleep.* New York: Free Press, 1996.

De Manacéine, Marie. *Sleep: Its Physiology, Pathology, Hygiene, and Psychology.* London: Walter Scott, Ltd., Paternoster Square, 1897.

Dement, William C. *Some Must Watch While Some Must Sleep.* New York: W. W. Norton & Company, 1978.

Diagnostic and Statistical Manual of Mental Disorders. 4th ed. Washington, D.C.: American Psychiatric Association, 1994.

Ferber, Richard, and Meir Kryger. *Principles and Practice of Sleep Medicine in the Child.* Philadelphia: W. B. Saunders Company, 1995.

Freud, Sigmund. *The Interpretation of Dreams.* Translated by A. A. Brill. New York: Gramercy Books, 1996.

Gray, Henry. *Gray's Anatomy.* New York: Gramercy Books, 1977.

Hammond, William Alexander. "On Sleep and Insomnia." *New York Medical Journal* (May 1865): 89–204.

———. *On Wakefulness.* Philadelphia: J. B. Lippincott & Co., 1866.

———. *Sleep and Its Derangements.* Philadelphia: J. B. Lippincott & Co., 1869.

Kleitman, Nathaniel. "Basic Rest-Activity Cycle—22 Years Later." *Sleep* 5, no. 4 (1982): 311–17.

———. Interview by Lynne Lamberg. APSS Conference, Nashville, Tenn., June 1989. Transcript provided by Lamberg.

———. *Sleep and Wakefulness: As Alternating Phases in the Cycle of Existence.* Chicago: University of Chicago Press, 1939.

———. *Sleep and Wakefulness.* Rev. and enlarged ed. Chicago: University of Chicago Press, 1963; Midway Reprint edition, 1987.

Kleitman, Nathaniel, F. J. Mullin, N. R. Cooperman, and S. Titelbaum. *Sleep Characteristics: How They Vary and React to Changing Conditions in the Group and the Individual.* Chicago: University of Chicago Press, 1937.

Kryger, Meir H., Thomas Roth, and William C. Dement. *Principles and Practice of Sleep Medicine.* 2nd ed. Philadelphia: W. B. Saunders Company, 1994.

Lamberg, Lynne. *Bodyrhythms: Chronobiology and Peak Performance.* New York: William Morrow and Company, 1994.

Lavie, Peretz. *The Enchanted World of Sleep.* Translated by Anthony Berris. New Haven: Yale University Press, 1996.

MacNish, Robert. *The Philosophy of Sleep.* 2nd ed. Hartford: S. Andrus and Son, 1844.

"1999 Omnibus Sleep in America Poll." National Sleep Foundation web site. March 27, 1999. <http://www.sleepfoundation.org/>.

Stopes, Marie Carmichael. *Sleep.* New York: Philosophical Library, 1956.

Thorpy, Michael J., and Jan Yager. *The Encyclopedia of Sleep and Sleep Disorders.* New York: Facts on File, 1991.

CHAPTER 1

Barbizet, Jacques. "Yawning." *Journal of Neurology, Neurosurgery, and Psychiatry* 21 (1958): 203–209.

Birnholz, Jason C. "The Development of Human Fetal Eye Movement Patterns." *Science* 213 (August 7, 1981): 679–81.

Dawes, G. S. "Breathing Before Birth in Animals and Man." *The New England Journal of Medicine* 290, no. 10 (March 7, 1974): 557–59.

Grant, Michael, and John Hazel. *Gods and Mortals in Classical Mythology.* Springfield, Mass.: G. & C. Merriam Company, 1973.

Hasan, Shabih U., et al. "Effect of Morphine on Breathing and Behavior in Fetal Sheep." *Journal of Applied Physiology* 64 (1988): 2058–65.

Kleitman, Nathaniel. "Studies on the Physiology of Sleep: The Effects of Prolonged Sleeplessness on Man." *American Journal of Physiology* 66 (1923): 67–92.

Rigatto, Henrique, et al. "Fetal Breathing and Behavior Measured Through a Double-Wall Plexiglas Window in Sheep." *Journal of Applied Physiology* 61 (1986): 160–64.

Sterman, M. B. "Relationship of Intrauterine Fetal Activity to Maternal Sleep Stage." *Experimental Neurology* 19 (1967): 98–106.

CHAPTER 2

Hall, Stephen S. "Our Memories, Our Selves." *The New York Times Magazine* (February 15, 1998): 26.

Kleitman, Nathaniel, and Theodore G. Engelmann. "Sleep Characteristics of Infants." *Journal of Applied Physiology* 6 (November 1953): 269–82.

Lawson, Robert W. "Blinking and Sleeping." *Nature* 165, no. 4185 (January 14, 1950): 81–82.

CHAPTER 3

Grotjahn, Martin. *My Favorite Patient: The Memoirs of a Psychoanalyst*. Frankfurt am Main: Verlag Peter Lang, 1987.

———. "The Process of Awakening." *The Psychoanalytic Review* 29, no. 1 (January 1942): 1–19.

Mavromatis, Andreas. *Hypnagogia: The Unique State of Consciousness Between Wakefulness and Sleep*. London: Routledge & Kegan Paul, 1987.

CHAPTER 4

Bernstein, Gail A., et al. "Caffeine Withdrawal in Normal School-Age Children." *Journal of the American Academy of Child and Adolescent Psychiatry* 37, no. 8 (August 1998): 858–65.

Curatolo, Peter W., and David Robertson. "The Health Consequences of Caffeine." *Annals of Internal Medicine* 98, no. 5 (May 1983): 641–51.

Higgins, Shaun O'L. *Measuring Spokane: A Numerical Look at a City and Its Region*. New Media Ventures, 1998.

Hollingworth, H. L. *The Influence of Caffein on Mental and Motor Efficiency*. New York: Science Press, 1912.

Kahn, E. J., Jr. "The Universal Drink." *The New Yorker* 34 and 35 (February 14, 21, and 28, and March 7, 1959).

Pendergrast, Mark. *For God, Country and Coca-Cola: The Unauthorized History of the Great American Soft Drink and the Company That Makes It.* New York: Collier Books, 1993.

Rehak, Melanie. "To Drink or Not to Drink." *The New York Times Magazine* (March 14, 1999): 20.

The Spokesman Review. Clippings dated January 22, 1953; May 24, 1953; July 17, 1955; July 18, 1955; November 7, 1963.

CHAPTER 5

Beldegreen, Alecia. *The Bed.* New York: Stewart, Tabori & Chang, 1991.

Brewer's Dictionary of Phrase & Fable. 15th ed. New York: Harper Collins, 1959.

Carter, Howard. *The Tomb of Tutankhamen.* New York: Excalibur Books/E. P. Dutton, 1972.

Close, Tim (Serta Mattress Co.). Telephone interview with author. San Francisco, December 9, 1998.

Green, Penelope. "The $2,300 Pillow and the Mass-Marketing of Luxury." *New York Times* (August 15, 1999): sec. 9–2.

Homer. *The Odyssey.* Translated by E. V. Rieu. Rev. ed. London: Penguin Books, 1991.

Jeffrey, Nancy Ann. "Sleep: The New Status Symbol." *Wall Street Journal* (April 2, 1999): W-1.

Kelly, Kevin, and Erin Jaeb. *Sleep on It!* Chicago: Children's Press, 1995.

McRoskey, Robert (McRoskey's Mattress Co.). Interview with author. San Francisco, October 7, 1998.

Purgavie, Dermot. "To Float, Perchance to Sleep." *San Francisco Examiner* (June 3, 1998): Z/A-1.

Reynolds, Reginald. *Beds.* New York: Doubleday & Company, 1951.

Rudofsky, Bernard. *Now I Lay Me Down to Eat: Notes and Footnotes on the Lost Art of Living.* Garden City, N.Y.: Anchor Books, 1980.

"Sleep." *Exploring* 21, no. 4 (winter 1997/98). Published by the Exploratorium, San Francisco.

Treasures of Tutankhamun. New York: Metropolitan Museum of Art, 1976.

Zipkin, Amy. "Counting Sheep and Dollar Signs." *New York Times* (May 31, 1998): 11.

CHAPTER 6

Bowers, Edwin F. "How Can We Get Enough Sleep?" *New York Medical Journal* 108 (August 3, 1918): 196.

Catechism of the Catholic Church. New York: Doubleday, 1995.

Central Intelligence Agency. Unsigned, declassified memorandum (March 18, 1953).

Edgar, Dale. Interview with author. Stanford University, Palo Alto, Calif., December 18, 1998.

Feeney, Susan. "Outwardly, Clinton Ignoring Fracas on the Hill." *San Francisco Examiner* (December 19, 1998): A-13.

Goode, Erica. "New Hope for the Losers in the Battle to Stay Awake." *New York Times* (November 3, 1998): D-1.

Haley, Bruce. *The Healthy Body and Victorian Culture*. Cambridge: Harvard University Press, 1978.

The Holy Bible. Revised Standard Version. New York: Meridian, 1974.

Johnson, H. M. "Is Sleep a Vicious Habit?" *Harper's* 157 (November 1928): 731.

Simpson, John. *The Concise Oxford Dictionary of Proverbs*. 2nd ed. Oxford: Oxford University Press, 1992.

Wills, Garry. *Saint Augustine*. New York: Viking Press, 1999.

CHAPTER 7

Abe, Kazuhiko, et al. "Sleepwalking and Recurrent Sleeptalking in Children of Childhood Sleepwalkers." *American Journal of Psychiatry* 141, no. 6 (June 1984): 800–801.

Aserinsky, Armond. Telephone interview with author. San Francisco, November 19, 1998.

Bates, Joah. "Posture During Sleep." *The Lancet* (February 7, 1942): 186.

Brody, Jane E. "Sleep-Related Violence." *New York Times on the Web,* January 16, 1996. July 31, 1997. <http://www.nytimes.com/>.

Broughton, Roger J. "Sleep Disorders: Disorders of Arousal?" *Science* 159 (March 8, 1968): 1070–78.

Broughton, Roger J., et al. "Homicidal Somnambulism: A Case Report." *Sleep* 17, no. 3 (1994): 253–64.

Broughton, Roger J., and Tetsuo Shimizu. "Sleep-Related Violence: A Medical and Forensic Challenge." *Sleep* 18, no. 9 (1995): 727–30.

Bucknill, John Charles, and Daniel Hack Tuke. *A Manual of Psychological Medicine.* 4th ed. Philadelphia: Lindsay and Blakiston, 1879.

Burns, J. C. "Curious Case of Somnambulism." *The Medical and Surgical Reporter* 32 (February 20, 1875): 158–59.

Cheever, John. "The Swimmer." *The Stories of John Cheever.* New York: Knopf, 1978.

Dunkell, Samuel. *Sleep Positions: The Night Language of the Body.* New York: William Morrow and Company, 1977.

Johnson, H. M., et al. "In What Positions Do Healthy People Sleep?" *Journal of the American Medical Association* 94, no. 26 (June 28, 1930): 2058–62.

Kelley, Matt. "Accused Killer Claims Sleepwalking." Associated Press, June 6, 1999. America Online: AOL News, June 7, 1999. <http://www.aol.com/>.

———. "Jury Convicts 'Sleepwalking' Husband." Associated Press, June 25, 1999. America Online: AOL News, June 25, 1999. <http://www.aol.com/>.

Kleitman, Nathaniel. Videotaped interview by Gerald Vogel, November 8, 1989. Videotape borrowed from UCLA School of Medicine, Brain Information Services, Los Angeles.

Kleitman, Nathaniel, et al. "Studies on the Physiology of Sleep: Motility and Body Temperature During Sleep." *American Journal of Physiology* 105 (1933): 574–84.

Kleitman, Nathaniel, and Hortense Kleitman. "The Sleep-Wakefulness Pattern in the Arctic." *The Scientific Monthly* 76, no. 6 (June 1953): 349–56.

Tuke, Daniel Hack. "Sleep-Walking and Hypnotism." London: J. & A. Churchill, 1884.

Yellowlees, D. "Homicide by a Somnambulist." *Journal of Mental Science* 24 (October 1878): 451–58.

CHAPTER 8

Abe, Kazuhiko, et al. "Sleepwalking and Recurrent Sleeptalking in Children of Childhood Sleepwalkers." *American Journal of Psychiatry* 141, no. 6 (June 1984): 800–801.

Arkin, Arthur M. "Sleep-Talking: A Review." *The Journal of Nervous and Mental Disease* 143, no. 2 (August 1966): 101–22.

———. *Sleep-Talking: Psychology and Psychophysiology.* Hillsdale, N.J.: Lawrence Erlbaum Associates, 1981.

Bixler, Edward O., et al. "Prevalence of Sleep Disorders in the Los Angeles Metropolitan Area." *American Journal of Psychiatry* 136, no. 10 (October 1979): 1257–62.

Burrell, Dwight R. "A Case of Sleep-Talking." *Proceedings of the American Medico-Psychological Association* (1904): 237–48.

Cook. T. W. "A Case of Abnormal Reproduction During Sleep." *The Journal of Abnormal and Social Psychology* 29 (1935): 465–70.

Ellman, Steven J. Telephone interview with author. San Francisco, September 14, 1999.

Freud, Sigmund. *The Origins of Psycho-Analysis: Letters to Wilhelm Fliess, Drafts and Notes: 1887–1902.* Edited by Marie Bonaparte, Anna Freud, Ernst Kris. New York: Basic Books, 1954.

Le Boeuf, Alan. "A Behavioral Treatment of Chronic Sleeptalking." *Journal of Behavior Therapy and Experimental Psychiatry* 10 (1979): 83–84.

McGregor, Dion. *Dion McGregor Dreams Again.* CD. Notes by Phil Milstein. New York: Tzadik Records, 1999.

———. *The Dream World of Dion McGregor.* New York: Bernard Geis Associates, 1964.

———. Radio interview from *The Long John Nebel Show,* July 8, 1964. Transcript available through the American Song-Poem Music Archives web site; link to "Dion McGregor Dreams Again." February 1999. <http://www.aspma.com/dion>.

Milstein, Phil. "Dion McGregor Dreams Again." American Song-

Poem Music Archives web site. February 1999. <http://www.aspma.com/dion>.

Pareja, Juan A., et al. "Native Language Shifts Across Sleep-Wake States in Bilingual Sleeptalkers." *Sleep* 22, no. 2 (March 15, 1999): 243–47.

Perlman, David. "Neanderthals Were Built to Talk." *San Francisco Chronicle* (April 28, 1998): A-5.

Strauss, Steven L. "A Sixty-Eight-Year-Old Man with Aphasia and Somniloquy." *Journal of Neurologic Rehabilitation* 10, no. 1 (1996): 53–54.

CHAPTER 9

Burr, Chandler. *A Separate Creation: The Search for the Biological Origins of Sexual Orientation*. New York: Hyperion, 1996.

Cartwright, Rosalind. "Social Psychology of Dream Reporting," Chap. 8 in *The Mind in Sleep: Psychology and Psychophysiology.* Hillsdale, N.J.: Lawrence Erlbaum Associates, 1978.

Cohen, Harvey D., and Arthur Shapiro. "Vaginal Blood Flow During Sleep." *Psychophysiology* 7, no. 2 (September 1970): 338.

Critchley, MacDonald. "Periodic Hypersomnia and Megaphagia in Adolescent Males." *Brain* 85, pt. 4 (December 1962): 627–57.

Fisher, Charles, et al. "Cycle of Penile Erection Synchronous With Dreaming (REM) Sleep." *Archives of General Psychiatry* 12 (January 1965): 29–45.

Goode, Erica. "Study Questions Gene Influence on Male Homosexuality." *New York Times* (April 23, 1999): A-19.

Karacan, I., et al. "The Clitoral Erection Cycle During Sleep." *Psychophysiology* 7, no. 2 (September 1970): 338.

———. "The Effect of Sexual Intercourse on Sleep Patterns and Nocturnal Penile Erections." *Psychophysiology* 7, no. 2 (September 1970): 338.

Kinsey, Alfred C. *Sexual Behavior in the Human Male*. Philadelphia: W. B. Saunders Company, 1948.

"Lawmakers Seek More Sleep for Pupils." *New York Times* (June 28, 1998): 19.

LeVay, Simon. *The Sexual Brain*. Cambridge: MIT Press, 1993.

Levin, Max. "Narcolepsy (Gélineau's Syndrome) and Other Varieties of Morbid Somnolence." *Archives of Neurology and Psychiatry* 22 (1929): 1172–1200.

Lucretius. *The Way Things Are.* Translated by Rolfe Humphries. Bloomington: Indiana University Press, 1968.

CHAPTER 10

Blakeslee, Sandra. "Surprising Theory on the Body Clock: Illuminate the Knee." *New York Times* (January 16, 1998): 1.

Blank, H. Robert. "Dreams of the Blind." *Psychoanalytic Quarterly* 27 (1958): 158–74.

Fuchs, Adalbert, and F. C. Wu. "Sleep With Half-Open Eyes (Physiologic Lagophthalmus)." *American Journal of Ophthalmology* 31 (1948): 717–20.

Hideshima, Ron. Interviews with author. San Francisco, April 5 and October 8, 1999.

Lamberg, Lynne. "Blind People Often Sleep Poorly; Research Shines Light on Therapy." *Journal of the American Medical Association* 280, no. 13 (October 7, 1998): 1123–26.

———. "Dawn's Early Light to Twilight's Last Gleaming." *Journal of the American Medical Association* 280, no. 18 (November 11, 1998): 1556–58.

Schiller, Francis. "Historical Note on Sleep and Eye Movements." *Sleep* 7, no. 3 (1984): 199–201.

CHAPTER 11

Brody, Jane E. "Fighting Jet Lag: A Battle Plan." *New York Times* (April 30, 1997): C-10.

Bryant, Samuel W. "What Jet Travel Does to Your Metabolic Clock." *Fortune* (November 1963): 160.

Ralph, Martin R., and Michael N. Lehman. "Transplantation: A New Tool in the Analysis of the Mammalian Hypothalamic Circadian Pacemaker." *Trends in Neuroscience* 14, no. 8 (1991): 362–66.

"Sleep & the Traveler." National Sleep Foundation web site. June 20, 1997. <http://www.sleepfoundation.org/>.

Von Frisch, Karl. *A Biologist Remembers.* Translated by Lisbeth Gombrich. Oxford: Pergamon Press, 1967.

———. *The Dancing Bees.* Translated by Dora Isle and Norman Walker. London: Methuen & Co., 1966.

Ward, Ritchie R. *Living Clocks.* New York: Knopf, 1971.

CHAPTER 12

Bird, Brian. "Pathological Sleep." *International Journal of Psychoanalysis* 35 (1954): 20–29.

"Chronic Fatigue Syndrome." National Institute of Allergy and Infectious Diseases web site. May 26, 1999. <http://www.niaid.nih.gov/>.

"Epstein-Barr Virus." Healthtouch Online. May 26, 1999. <http://www.healthtouch.com/>.

Freud, Sigmund. *Collected Papers.* Vol. 4. Translated by Joan Riviere. London: Hogarth Press, 1934.

Greenberg, Brigitte. "Study Traces Causes of Car Crashes." Associated Press, December 21, 1999. America Online: AOL News, December 21, 1999. <http://www.aol.com/>.

Grmek, Mirko D. *History of AIDS.* Translated by Russell C. Maulitz and Jacalyn Duffin. Princeton: Princeton University Press, 1991.

Jablon, Robert. "Obesity on the Rise in the U.S." Associated Press, October 26, 1999. America Online: AOL News, October 26, 1999. <http://www.aol.com/>.

Johnson, Glen. "New Campaign Targets Drowsy Drivers." Associated Press, June 3, 1999. America Online: AOL News, June 3, 1999. <http://www.aol.com/>.

Lavie, Peretz. "The Touch of Morpheus: Pre–20th Century Accounts of Sleepy Patients." *Neurology* 41 (November 1991): 1841–44.

"New York Neurological Society, Meeting, May 6, 1884." *Journal of Nervous and Mental Disease* 11 (1884): 613–18.

"*Pneumocystis* Pneumonia—Los Angeles." *Morbidity and Mortality Weekly Report* 30, no. 21 (June 5, 1981): 250–52.

Schlossberg, David, ed. *Infectious Mononucleosis.* 2nd ed. New York: Springer-Verlag, 1989.

Shilts, Randy. *And the Band Played On.* New York: St. Martin's Press, 1987.

Willey, Malcolm M. "The Psychic Utility of Sleep." *Journal of Abnormal Psychology and Social Psychology* 19 (1924): 174–78.

———. "Sleep as an Escape Mechanism." *Psychoanalytic Review* 11 (1924): 181–83.

CHAPTER 13

Calkins, Mary Whiton. "Statistics of Dreams." *The American Journal of Psychology* 5, no. 3 (1893): 311–43.

Frazer, James. *The Golden Bough.* Abr. ed. New York: Penguin Books, 1996.

Germain, Anne, et al. "Variations in the Physiological Correlates of Dream Recall Across REM Episodes." *Sleep* 22, suppl. 1 (April 15, 1999): S-176.

Greene, Graham. *A World of My Own: A Dream Diary.* New York: Viking Penguin, 1994.

Jouvet, Michel. *The Paradox of Sleep: The Story of Dreaming.* Translated by Laurence Garey. Cambridge, Mass.: A Bradford Book, MIT, 1999.

Kleitman, Nathaniel. "Patterns of Dreaming." *Scientific American* (November 1960): 82–88.

Lavie, Peretz, ed. "History of Sleep Research." *World Federation of Sleep Research Societies Newsletter* web site, vol. 5, no. 1 (1996). <http://www.wfsrs.org/newsletter.html>.

Rupp, Rebecca. *Committed to Memory: How We Remember and Why We Forget.* New York: Crown Publishers, 1998.

CHAPTER 14

Berg, Nancy. Telephone interview with author. San Francisco, August 24, 1999.

Blustein, Bonnie Ellen. "The Brief Career of 'Cerebral Hyperaemia': William A. Hammond and His Insomniac Patients, 1854–90." *Journal of the History of Medicine and Allied Sciences* 41, no. 1 (January 1986): 24–51.

———. *Preserve Your Love for Science: Life of William A. Hammond,*

American Neurologist. Cambridge: Cambridge University Press, 1991.

Breggin, Peter R. "Halcion Malpractice Case Won in Court." Center for the Study of Psychiatry and Psychology web site. August 14, 1999. <http://www.breggin.com/>.

"Critic: FDA Withholding Data on Controversial Sleeping Pill." CNN Interactive, May 23, 1996. August 14, 1999. <http://www.cnn.com/>.

"FDA and the Ongoing Ban of Tryptophan." Smart Basics web site. November 13, 1999. <http://www.smartbasics.com/>.

"FDA Seeks Justice Probe of Halcion Sleeping Pill." CNN Interactive, May 31, 1996. August 14, 1999. <http://www.cnn.com/>.

Galewitz, Phil. "Mid-Night Sleeping Pill Developed." Associated Press, August 10, 1999. America Online: AOL News, August 11, 1999. <http://www.aol.com/>.

Hammond, William Alexander. "Why We Sleep." *Appleton's Journal* 1, no. 1 (April 3, 1869): 14–15.

"Impurities Confirmed in Dietary Supplement 5-Hydroxy-L-Tryptophan." Food and Drug Administration web site, August 31, 1998. November 13, 1999. <http://www.fda.gov/>.

"New York Neurological Society, Meeting of October 7th, 1890." *The Journal of Nervous and Mental Disease* 15 (1890): 760–66.

Styron, William. *Darkness Visible: A Memoir of Madness*. New York: Random House, 1990.

Tuke, Daniel Hack, ed. *A Dictionary of Psychological Medicine*. London: J. & A. Churchill, 1892.

Winslow, Forbes. *On Obscure Diseases of the Brain and Disorders of the Mind*. Philadelphia: Blanchard & Lea, 1860.

CHAPTER 15

Blakeslee, Sandra. "Mystery of Sleep Yields As Studies Reveal Immune Tie." *New York Times* (August 3, 1993): B-5.

Darko, Denis F., et al. "Fatigue, Sleep Disturbance, Disability, and Indices of Progression of HIV Infection." *American Journal of Psychiatry* 149, no. 4 (April 1992): 514–20.

———. "Growth Hormone, Fatigue, Poor Sleep, and Disability in

HIV Infection." *Neuroendocrinology* 67 (1998): 317–24.

———. "Sleep Electroencephalogram . . . and Human Immunodeficiency Virus Infection." *Proceedings of the National Academy of Sciences, U.S.A.* 92 (December 1995): 12080–84.

Poscher, Margaret. Interview with author. San Francisco, September 23, 1999.

Smolensky, Michael and Lynne Lamberg. *The Body Clock Guide to Better Health.* New York: Henry Holt & Co., 2000.

CHAPTER 16

Borges, Jorge Luis. *Selected Poems.* Edited by Alexander Coleman. New York: Viking Penguin, 1999.

"Bovine Spongiform Encephalopathy (BSE)." World Health Organization web site, November 1996. November 10, 1999. <http://www.who.int/>.

"Bovine Spongiform Encephalopathy ('Mad Cow Disease')." University of Illinois at Urbana-Champaign ACES web site. November 10, 1999. <http://w3.aces.uiuc.edu/>.

Gambetti, Pierluigi. "Insomnia in Prion Diseases: Sporadic and Familial." *The New England Journal of Medicine* 340, no. 21 (May 27, 1999): 1675–77.

Guilleminault, Christian, et al. *Fatal Familial Insomnia: Inherited Prion Diseases, Sleep, and the Thalamus.* New York: Raven Press, 1994.

Lugaresi, Elio, et al. "Fatal Familial Insomnia and Dysautonomia with Selective Degeneration of Thalamic Nuclei." *The New England Journal of Medicine* 315, no. 16 (October 16, 1986): 997–1003.

Mastrianni, James A., et al. "Prion Protein Conformation in a Patient with Sporadic Fatal Insomnia." *The New England Journal of Medicine* 340, no. 21 (May 27, 1999): 1630–38.

Webster, Katharine. "Form of Fatal Insomnia Discovered." Associated Press, May 26, 1999. America Online: AOL News, May 26, 1999. <http://www.aol.com/>.

Yoder, Robert M. "So You Think You Need Eight Hours' Sleep!" *Saturday Evening Post* 229 (April 6, 1957): 42.

CHAPTER 17

Gilmore, Rhonda (pseudonym). Telephone interview with author. San Francisco, June 1, 1999.

Villalba, Constanza. "Guys Aren't Alone in Sawing Logs at Night." *New York Times* (June 13, 1999): WH-23.

CHAPTER 18

"Abstracts of 13th Annual Meeting of the Associated Professional Sleep Societies, June 19–24, 1999." *Sleep* 22, suppl. 1 (April 15, 1999).

Askew, Judith Stiles, ed. *Menopause News* 6, no. 1 (January/February 1996).

Carlson, A. J., N. Kleitman, C. W. Muehlberger, F. C. McLean, H. Gullicksen, and R. B. Carlson. *Studies on the Possible Intoxicating Action of 3.2 Per Cent Beer.* Chicago: University of Chicago Press, 1934.

Cheng, Vicki. "Nathaniel Kleitman, Sleep Expert, Dies at 104." *New York Times* (August 19, 1999): C-26.

Kolata, Gina. "The Fat War: Hope Amid the Harm." *New York Times* (October 31, 1999): sec. 4-1.

McCarley, Robert, et al. "A Year in Review." Course book for APSS conference seminar "A Year in Review," June 20, 1999.

Neergaard, Lauran. "Study Examines Age-Melatonin Link." Associated Press, November 5, 1999. America Online: AOL News, November 5, 1999. <http://www.aol.com/>.

INDEX

A

adolescents. *See also* children
    Kleine-Levin syndrome,
        155–56
    wet dreams, 148–50
Ahasuerus, King, 80
Alcmaeon, 7
Ambien, 234–35, 309, 310
Anatomy of Sleep; or, The Art of
    Procuring Sound and Re-
    freshing Slumber at Will
    (Binns), 84–85, 89–90,
    236–37
Ancoli-Israel, Sonia, 307–308
apnea. *See* obstructive sleep
    apnea syndrome (OSAS)
Aristophanes, 80

Aristotle, 7, 19, 213
Arkin, Arthur M., 134–39
Aserinsky, Armond, 162, 224
    experiments with father,
        117–20
    REM sleep demonstration,
        170–71
Aserinsky, Eugene, 22–25,
    146–47, 312
    dreaming and REM sleep,
        164–65
    experiments with son, 117–20
    infant blinking study, 22–24
    nightmares, 223–24
    precedents for REM sleep
        theory, 163–64